# LOSE WEIGHT

# *FAST*

# Diet

Dedicated to the millions of people who are committed to losing weight. May you live a happy and healthy life.

## By Alex A. Lluch
### Health and Fitness Expert &
### Author of Over 4 Million Books Sold!

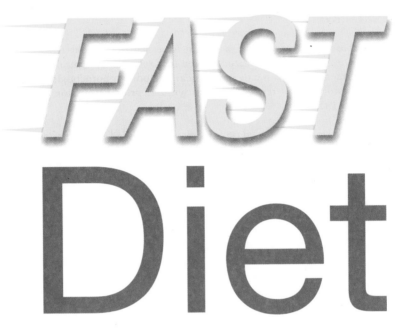

**WS** Publishing Group 📖
www.WSPublishingGroup.com
San Diego, California

# Lose Weight Fast Diet

## By Alex A. Lluch

Copyright © 2012 WS Publishing Group, Inc.
San Diego, California 92128

Nutritional and fitness guidelines based on information provided by the United States Food and Drug Administration, Food and Nutrition Information Center, National Agricultural Library, Agricultural Research Service, and the U.S. Department of Agriculture.

For more best-selling titles by WS Publishing Group,
visit www.wspublishinggroup.com

Photographer:
Nathaniel Kam, www.nathanielkamphotography.com

Models:
Lauren Jackson, www.laurenrjackson.com
Leonardo Cerqueira, www.modelmayhem.com/1013282

Meal Plan:
Lindsey Toth, MS, RD, www.lindseytoth.com
734.216.0004

Image Credit:
© iStockphoto/stdemi (fruit & vegetables)

ISBN: 978-1-936061-38-9

Printed in China

# contents

# contents

# Introduction

You know the frightening statistics by now: 67 percent of Americans are overweight, and 34 percent are considered obese. Millions of people are struggling with their weight every day and suffering the effects, from lack of energy to infertility to diabetes to heart disease. Perhaps most tangible, however, are the feelings of frustration, disappointment, and self-doubt that trying to lose weight and failing bring.

That's because so many diets are doomed to fail. They either force you to go cold turkey with the foods you love (causing cravings and bingeing), tell you to substitute real food with an unappealing powdered drink or meal replacement bar, or promote fast and easy weight loss through eating only certain foods and eliminating whole food groups (re: the lemonade-and-cayenne pepper diet or the grapefruit diet; extremely unhealthy). None of these types of diets are healthy or sustainable, meaning you'll only gain the weight right back afterward. And you're not learning any new eating or exercise habits, so you'll simply revert back to your old lifestyle, the one that made you gain weight in the first place.

The *Lose Weight Fast Diet*, however, is full of the most powerful, proven secrets in the world to help you lose the weight you want in record time. Slim down for a class reunion, vacation, birthday celebration, or just because swimsuit season is never far off. Or maybe there's no special occasion; maybe you're just tired of carrying around 10 or more extra pounds and you know, with dedication and several fast lifestyle changes, you can be at weight you want. Being healthier, happier, and in better shape with more energy are always the best reasons for losing weight. Medical research has shown that losing just 5 to 10 percent of your body weight can significantly improve a person's health by lowering cholesterol and the risk of heart disease, stroke, and diabetes.

Losing weight is never easy. As we age and our metabolisms slow down, the body gets comfortable with the extra pounds, and it's tougher to lose them. Your body needs a jump-start, just like a car with a stalled battery! You'll find the diet and fitness tips in this book to be just what you need to get moving more efficiently, cooking smarter, planning ahead, and eating better. And unlike other weight-loss plans, where you're eliminating the nutrients your body truly needs, you won't be starving or exhausted. This program is what is considered a "flexible diet," one that instructs people to monitor the consumption of calories to lose weight. You won't starve, eat only one kind of food, or miss out on dinners with friends or your favorite treats — you just need to implement the diet and fitness secrets you'll learn in this book and keep your eye on the prize — losing weight, body fat, and inches!

The heart of the *Lose Weight Fast Diet* includes three basic steps:

1. Using a formula to determine the calories your body burns at rest, or your BMR.

2. Tracking everything you eat and all the physical activity you perform daily.

3. Creating a substantial daily calorie deficit — meaning that you are expending more calories than you take in through a combination of eating less and burning calories with exercise. The larger the calorie deficit you create each day, the more weight you will lose.

At the end of each day, you will add up the calories you ate and drank. Then you'll take the resulting number and subtract the calories burned from physical activity to calculate your Net Calories. Next, subtract your BMR (the calories your body burns at rest) to find your daily total calorie deficit. You can find a detailed example of this formula in the section called "Journal Pages."

In addition, with this program you will mentally create a calorie "budget" for each meal and snack, which means anticipating how many calories you need to save and preparing for each meal with a set amount to spend in mind. For example, you might budget 400 calories for lunch. You can have any meal and drink you want, as long as you stay within your budget. And, if it's possible to save a few calories by eating less than the budgeted amount, you can save up for the next meal or do slightly less exercise to lose even more weight!

If it sounds like a big change and hard work, that's because it is. No one is going to pretend it will be easy. You will have to make major changes, like cutting out empty carbs and calories, eating more fruits, vegetables, and whole grains, and building fitness into your life every day. But the results will be worth it. Fitting into that favorite dress again, seeing the look on an old boyfriend's face, lounging on the beach in a swimsuit without feeling anxious — you will be highly rewarded for your hard work over the next few weeks and beyond.

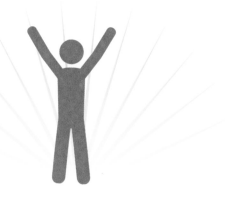

By purchasing this book, you have taken the first step in your weight-loss journey to looking and feeling amazing!

# How to Use This Book

**Congratulations! You've taken the first step** toward losing real weight in a short amount of time by getting all the tools you need. Simply eating less, making a few foods swaps, or spending some extra time at the gym isn't going to allow you to lose weight in a short amount of time. People who think they can lose considerable weight without any help get frustrated and fail. This book offers you many valuable tools and features for cutting calories, getting in great shape, and successfully meeting your weight-loss goals, including:

## Filling out your personal health and fitness profile

Before you begin the *Lose Weight Fast Diet* program, you need to build Your Personal Profile. This section helps you assess your current physical state, habits, and preferences for diet and exercise. With this information, you will be able to determine where you started and how far you've come, as well as identify your goals and any potential obstacles.

In this section you will also determine the optimum amount of calories, fat, and carbs that you will aim to eat every day.

## Determining your BMR and creating a daily calorie deficit

An important part of the *Lose Weight Fast Diet* program is calculating your basal metabolic rate, or BMR. Your BMR is the number of calories your body would burn naturally, even if you didn't move all day. Knowing this number is the first step to this program because it's how you build a calorie deficit.

Each day, you will total up the amount of calories you have eaten and subtract the calories you have burned from physical activity to find your Net Calorie Total. In order to lose weight, you need to create a substantial calorie deficit each day, through a combination of diet and exercise. For example, one day, you may be able to cut 500 calories out of your diet, and then also burn 500 calories through exercise to create a 1,000 calorie deficit. Once you create a 3,500 calorie deficit, you will have lost 1 pound.

## Powerful diet secrets and tips, fast places to trim calories, motivational quotes, and more

Each chapter and section of this book is packed with the secrets of cutting calories, making lifestyle changes, and losing weight. You will learn to boost your metabolism, make healthier eating decisions, as well as one of the best weight-loss strategies around: developing a game plan for avoiding pitfalls and sticking to your daily calorie goals. Through this book, you will practice conscious eating, curb your appetite, and stop sabotaging your weight-loss efforts. You will also learn to anticipate and recognize situations that cause you to binge or eat unhealthy foods, and pinpoint the emotions and triggers that cause you to overeat.

You will recognize the changes you can make without starving or depriving yourself, because no diet and fitness plan is going to work if you're feeling lethargic and hungry all the time. Burning hundreds of calories more than you take in a day might sound difficult, and that's why each chapter in this book is complete with "Did You Know" facts, motivational quotes, as well as quick and easy places to trim 100, 200, and 300 or more calories. You'll discover new ways to eat less and lose weight that you never even thought of!

Finally, the diet section ends with 100 at-a-glance principles for losing weight. Any time you need a quick reminder for how to eat smart, make healthy diet swaps, or maintain motivation, flip back to this section to read the diet secrets at-a-glance.

## Ultimate fitness secrets for burning calories and body fat and staying motivated

Fitness is going to be the second key to losing weight in a short amount of time. You can't do it with diet alone! These chapters will give you all the tips, tricks and tools to maximize each and every workout and physical activity you perform. You'll get insight into everything from fitness basics to little-known secrets of getting in shape quickly and without burning out.

In the Activities & Calories Burned chapter, you'll see that calories are burned in all sorts of ways, from sports to casual physical activity to normal household chores. This section that will be a great asset in finding the sports and activities that you can make a part of your daily routine to burn calories.

## Powerful exercise program for maximum weight loss

The fitness section also includes a detailed exercise program that combines strength training with a cardio circuit six days out of the week to burn calories and body fat quickly. You will switch off each day between an upper body, lower body, and core strength training circuit. Each day, you will also engage in a cardio plan. This book includes two custom cardio programs — a running workout and a walking workout. Or you can choose your own cardio activity, such as hiking, aerobics, and more. The last day of the week is to rest, recuperate, and relax.

Finally, the fitness section ends with at-a-glance secrets for exercise and living an active, healthy life. The goal is to make physical activity a part of your everyday routine — something you even look forward to. Refer to the secrets for getting fit in this section when you need a reminder of how to incorporate exercise and fitness into your day.

## Reusable grocery list of healthy foods

Stop wandering the aisles of the supermarket, wondering what to buy to keep you and your family eating right. The *Lose Weight Fast Diet* grocery list in the front of the book tears out to bring to the store and is laminated so it can be used again and again with a dry-erase marker.

This list takes the guesswork out of shopping by providing you with a comprehensive list of healthy, weight-loss-smart products and food items by category — everything from fresh and canned produce to beverages to sweet treats! You can even write in your own supermarket favorites as you discover them. Even with this helpful list, don't forget to read the nutritional labels on all products.

## Follow the *Lose Weight Fast* custom meal plan from dietitian Lindsey Toth

The *Lose Weight Fast Diet* meal plan lets you enjoy the foods you love without the added fat or calories. Lindsey Toth, registered dietitian and advisor to PepsiCo's Global Nutrition Communications department, created a custom meal plan for the *Lose Weight Fast Diet* that includes 20 original breakfasts, 20 lunches, and 20 dinners that can be mixed and matched for smart eating throughout the day. Each meal contains a balance of carbohydrates, healthy fats, protein, and fiber to help you slim down, have tons of energy, and feel satiated after each meal. A list of weight-loss friendly snacks is also included.

Eating from the meal plan means never having to guess about the nutritional values of an item, and makes recording your intake in your diet journal that much easier. Plus, the meals are simple and delicious, so anyone can follow the recipes and enjoy a well-balanced dish at every meal.

## Use your number one weight-loss tool!

People who keep a food and fitness journal are proven to lose *twice* as much weight as those who don't. As you read all the valuable, powerful weight-loss and fitness tips in this book, you will be keeping track of what you eat and drink in the journal in the back of the book. Each daily page lets you write down the food and beverages you consume daily, as well as the physical activities you perform to burn calories. You'll easily be able to see what you've eaten and, thus, plan ahead for each meal and workout.

Keeping a diet journal will most likely be a healthy reality check. Studies have shown that people tend to dramatically underestimate the number of calories in the foods they eat — by as much as 50 percent! The diet and fitness journal portion of this book allows you to break down your caloric intake by meal and item to get real about exactly how many calories you're consuming. Once you recognize the high-calorie foods in your diet, you can replace some things with lower calorie options or cut back on portion sizes. Additionally, having your food intake right in front of you keeps you accountable — because who wants to look back and see the hundreds of calories from a pizza-and-cheese-bread binge written in their journal? You'll think twice before indulging in a huge or highly caloric meal. The journal will also help keep you motivated to exercise daily and provide a place to record your weight as the numbers on the scale begin to drop.

## What happens after you lose weight?

Fast-forward a few weeks and you've lost 5, 10, 20 or more pounds by following the diet and exercise program in this book! Now what? You can't just fall back into your old habits. You've worked too hard to put the weight right back on. This chapter gives you the secrets to making long-lasting changes that make exercising and eating smart a *lifestyle* and not just a short-term weight-loss experience. And every time you need a reminder of the best, most proven ways to be healthy, have energy, and make smart food choices, you should refer back to this book. Keep using a diet and fitness journal, your healthy eating grocery list, the meal plan, and the secrets in this book to keep dropping unwanted pounds.

If you're looking for a larger diet journal following the end of this program, the *Lose Weight Fast Diet Journal* is the companion journal to this book, and contains 30 weeks of space to record daily food and water intake, physical activity, energy levels, servings from each food group, goals, achievements, and much more.

## Nutritional information for more than 1,000 foods right at your fingertips!

Do you know how many calories are in your banana, egg salad, or glass of wine? Probably not, but the Nutrition Facts section in the back of this book will allow you to look up the calories, fat, carbs, protein and fiber for more than 1,000 common food items. Transfer these amounts into your diet journal to accurately keep track of your daily intake.

# Your Personal
# Profile

**Begin your program by** gathering some information to assess your current physical state, habits, and preferences.

Fill in the information on the following pages. Visit your primary care physician and have your cholesterol, triglycerides, and blood pressure measured. These levels will also factor into the choices you make when creating your diet and fitness plan. You should also take your current measurements and place a "Before" photo in this section. It will be motivating to look back and see a visual of where you began and how far you have come.

Next, assess your diet and fitness history. You will also answer some questions about your past attempts to lose weight and what obstacles you encountered. Finally, outline your goals. Determine what you hope to accomplish with this program, which types of physical activities you most enjoy, and your intake goals, including the specific amounts of calories, fats, and carbs your diet should include daily.

Good luck meeting all your goals!

## Your Health Profile

Complete the following personal health profile. You can request necessary information from your primary health care provider.

Name:_____          Triglycerides:_____

Age:_____          HDL Cholesterol:_____

Height:_____          LDL Cholesterol:_____

Total cholesterol:_____          Blood Pressure:_____


Current Physical Activity: (sedentary, moderately active, very active)

_____

_____

_____

_____

_____

Current Diet & Eating Habits: (fast food, snack often, late night eating, etc.)

_____

_____

_____

_____

Other Current Habits: (smoking, drinking, lack of sleep, etc.)

_____

_____

_____

_____

_____

_____

DATE:_____     WEIGHT:_____     BODY FAT %:_____

**MEASUREMENTS:**

[     ] chest     [     ] biceps     [     ] waist     [     ] hips     [     ] thighs

tape your photo here

PHOTO COMMENTS:_____

## Dietary Habits Questionnaire

The following questions will assist you in developing your weight-loss program.

**Which best describes your daily eating habits?**
❑ Three average meals
❑ Graze frequently
❑ One large meal, little else

**What types of food do you crave the most?**
❑ Meat/fish
❑ Fruit/vegetables
❑ Bread/cereals/rice
❑ Sweets

**Do you typically eat out or prepare food for yourself?**
❑ I usually cook my food
❑ I eat out or have pre-made meals

**What is your weight-loss goal?**
❑ Lose 10 or more pounds
❑ Maintain weight
❑ Lose a little weight
❑ Improve health

**Which habits do you have?**
❑ Skipping meals
❑ Drinking full-sugar soda
❑ Carb addiction
❑ Overeating while dining out

**Describe your body type:**
❑ Overweight
❑ Average
❑ Muscular

**For what particular event (if any) do you want to lose weight?**

_____

_____

_____

_____

_____

_____

**What is your number one reason for wanting to lose weight?**

_____

_____

_____

_____

_____

## Your Diet & Intake Goals

A huge part of your weight-loss journey will be managing your diet and intake. Record your goals here and use them as a barometer for what you eat every day.

---

**YOUR DIET GOALS**

_____

_____

_____

_____

_____

_____

_____

---

**YOUR INTAKE GOALS**

Based on the number of calories your diet allows, list the daily targets that you would like to meet. (Your primary care physician can also help you determine the appropriate amounts.)

**DAILY CALORIES:**          **FAT gms:**          **CARBS gms:**          **OTHER:** _____

**NOTES:** _____

_____

_____

_____

_____

_____

## Your Fitness History

It is important to look back at your past experiences with getting in shape and losing weight to determine the diet and workout plan that will have the greatest chance for success.

Is there any reason why you should not engage in physical activity?

_____

At what age were you in your best physical shape?

_____

Have you ever participated in a workout program? When?

_____

How long did you stay with the program?

_____

What did the program include?

_____

What led you to or inspired you to get into shape now?

_____

What obstacles have kept you from meeting your fitness goals?

_____

What will ensure these obstacles do not inhibit you this time?

_____

Rate your current fitness level on a scale of 1-10 (1=Worst 10=Best).

_____

## Workout Plan Questionnaire

A successful fitness plan is one that includes activities you enjoy. Be honest in answering the following questions and you will be able to develop a plan you can maintain.

Which types of physical activity do you enjoy participating in?

❑ Aerobics
❑ Active gardening
❑ Backpacking
❑ Baseball/softball
❑ Bicycling/spinning
❑ Climbing
❑ Cross country skiing
❑ Dancing
❑ Downhill skiing
❑ Football
❑ Golfing
❑ Hiking
❑ Hockey
❑ Jogging/running
❑ Jump roping

❑ Martial arts
❑ Pilates
❑ Racquetball/handball
❑ Roller blading
❑ Rowing
❑ Soccer
❑ Skating
❑ Stair/bench stepping
❑ Stretching
❑ Swimming
❑ Tennis
❑ Volleyball
❑ Walking
❑ Weight training
❑ Yoga

**How many times a week do you want to work out?**

❑   1-2 days   ❑   2-3 days   ❑   3-4 days   ❑   5+ days

**How long will each session be, on average?**

❑ 10-20 minutes
❑ 20-30 minutes
❑ 30-45 minutes

❑ 45-60 minutes
❑ 60-90 minutes
❑ 90+ minutes

## Your Fitness Goals

By first identifying your goals, you can create a specific workout routine to help you achieve them. Your goals should be specific, quantifiable, realistic, and time-based. Fill out the following questions honestly and with a critical eye. You'll be able to use the resulting information to get inspired and ward off possible pitfalls.

What do you want to accomplish with your workout program?
(Check the boxes next to the goals that are most important to you.)

❏ Improve cardiovascular fitness and endurance

❏ Improve diet and/or eating habits

❏ Improve flexibility

❏ Improve health

❏ Improve strength

❏ Improve muscle tone and shape

❏ Increase energy

❏ Lose weight

❏ Prevent injury and/or rehabilitate injury

❏ Train for a sports-specific event

❏ Reduce cholesterol

❏ Reduce blood pressure

❏ Reduce risk of disease

❏ Reduce stress

❏ Gain weight

❏ Other: _____

❏ Other: _____

What types of physical activity do you like and dislike?

_____

_____

_____

_____

Do you prefer to exercise alone, with a partner, or in a group?

_____

_____

_____

_____

## Calculating Your BMR

Knowing your basal metabolic rate, or BMR, is crucial to this program. Your BMR is the number of calories your body burns naturally, at rest. Your BMR is based on your age, height, and current weight and decreases with age, meaning that it becomes harder to lose weight and keep it off as you get older. However, with a healthy diet and fitness plan, you can increase your BMR and lose weight more easily.

Use these formulas to calculate your BMR, then use this number in your daily diet and fitness journal pages.

Female BMR = 655 + (4.3 x weight in pounds) + (4.7 x height in inches) - (4.7 x age in years)

Male BMR = 66 + (6.3 x weight in pounds) + (12.9 x height in inches) - (6.8 x age in years)

Your BMR:

# Chapter 01

"The great thing in the world is not
so much where we stand, as in what
direction we are moving."

~ Oliver Wendell Holmes

# Changing the Way You Live

**Losing weight takes a tremendous effort.** If it were easy, everyone would be at their perfect weight. When you talk about a body and lifestyle makeover, you can feel yourself getting excited, but when it comes time to actually implement the changes, your to-do list feels so long that you get overwhelmed and give up. Or in the past you might have made it a few weeks into a weight-loss plan, failed to see results, and quit. It's natural for the body to resist change. Your body tries to protect itself by slowing its basal metabolism, the rate at which you burn calories at rest, making weight loss difficult. However, this program will have you looking and feeling better immediately, starting with the simple lifestyle changes in the chapter. Read through them and commit yourself to implementing them. They are what your body and mind need to jump-start your weight loss, give you more energy, and get you motivated to complete the program.

Mahatma Gandhi once said, "Be the change you want to see in the world." Being healthier and living better are goals everyone should strive for. You will likely find that after living the *Lose Weight Fast Diet* program, you won't want to stop! You'll feel better and slimmer than ever before, and you won't want to go back to old habits that packed on the extra pounds. However, even if you don't continue beyond this program, know that all the changes you'll find in this book are sustainable for a lifetime. This book gives you the tools to lose real weight in 4 weeks or less, including powerful, proven diet and exercise secrets and tips, motivational quotes, a healthy eating shopping list, healthy meal plan, nutrition facts for common foods, and, the ultimate weight-loss tool, a daily diet and fitness journal. With all this at your fingertips, it's just up to you to put everything into practice.

Losing weight quickly starts by modifying your everyday habits. Today, you get a clean slate to erase the past and create a new, healthier, thinner way of living.

## Keep your eye on the prize

Staying motivated is all about determining the top reasons you want and need to lose weight, and reminding yourself on the days you're tempted to eat a high-calorie dessert or skip the gym. Are you losing weight to look and feel great at a special event that is a few weeks away, such as a high school reunion, wedding, vacation, or birthday? Did your doctor advise you that losing 10 pounds will help reduce your risk of disease, lower your blood pressure, or help you get pregnant? Are you looking forward to the increased amount of energy you'll have after losing extra weight? Or are you simply tired of feeling powerless to food? Make a short list of the top 3 reasons you are losing weight. Hang this list where you can see it every day to remind you, along with a motivational image — a gorgeous beach, a dress you'd like to buy in a smaller size, the hike you plan to take when you have more energy.

## Create great new habits

Changing the way you live starts with building new, healthy habits that support your weight loss. One interesting benefit that men have over women when it comes to changing the way they live is that men tend to zone in on a single task, whereas the female brain approaches goals from a broader perspective, often making it more difficult to accomplish every task. No matter your gender, focus on your biggest problems first, be it that late night eating, fried food, or overeating when dining out with friends.

Let's say you have the bad habit of overeating at lunch, leaving you overfull and sluggish all afternoon. Chances are, you're skipping breakfast (no, coffee is not breakfast) or having empty carbs in the morning (such as a bagel or croissant). What you need, instead, is a protein and fiber-filled meal that jump-starts your metabolism and mind, and prevents overeating throughout the day. Try having whole grains, such as wheat toast or instant oatmeal, with 2 hardboiled eggs and a piece of fruit or low-fat yogurt. Or if you have more time in the morning, whip up a vegetable omelette with an English muffin on the side.

This book gives you the tools to lose weight fast, including powerful, proven diet and exercise secrets and tips, motivational quotes, a healthy eating shopping list, healthy meal plan, nutrition facts for common foods, and, the ultimate weight-loss tool, a daily diet and fitness journal.

Get in the habit of keeping healthy breakfast ingredients in your kitchen or fridge at work, and you'll have made one awesome, positive change to your lifestyle. Focus on including the good behavior into your routine every day for a week until it becomes second nature.

## Eat from all 6 of the main food groups

There are 6 main food groups: grains, fruits, vegetables, dairy, meat and beans, and oils and sweets. Odds are, you've been overdoing it in some and avoiding others all together. For instance, less than 3.5 percent of American men and women eat the FDA-recommended amount of fruits and vegetables. Unfortunately, when food groups are short-changed, you do not receive the balance of protein, carbohydrates, and plant-based nutrients that your body needs. To kick-start a sluggish metabolism, maintain your energy and inspire the body to burn fat cells, you must eat a balanced diet. The better you eat, the better your body works and the faster you'll lose weight. And you'll find that it only takes a few short days for your body to stop craving fatty and sugary processed foods. Some foods that pack mega-nutrients include low-fat yogurt, spinach, salmon, berries, avocados, whole grains, bell peppers, and olive oil.

### Did You Know?

Depending on your height and body fat percentage, losing 10 pounds could mean dropping as many as 2 clothing sizes!

## Ransack your kitchen and pantry

Step 1: Get a big trash bag. Step 2: Open your cabinets, pantry, fridge and yes, even the hidden spots where you stash treats. Step 3: Throw every high-calorie, high-fat, sugary, salty, processed piece of food into your trash bag. Step 4: Take one last look in the bag before you toss it into a dumpster. Say goodbye to unhealthy, bloating, weight-gain-causing snacks and treats! Step 5: Feel inspired by your spotless (perhaps nearly empty) cupboards and shelves. You now have a clean slate to start filling your kitchen with healthy foods. Likewise, cravings are very visual, so if you open your cupboards and don't see fatty foods, you won't constantly think about them.

## Break the addiction to high-calorie food!

Did you realize that constantly treating yourself to high-calorie foods can lead to an actual addiction to them? Eating a high-calorie meal triggers the release of dopamine and other feel-good chemicals in the brain. However, a ground-breaking report from the 2009 meeting for the Society for Neuroscience showed that rats that were fed a high-calorie diet of items like bacon, sausage, and cheesecake actually had diminished responses in the pleasure centers of their brains over time. As the animals' brain reward circuits became less responsive, they continued to overeat and become more and more obese. Their brains actually began to mimic those of rats addicted to drugs as they became addicted to high-calorie foods! Break this cycle by eliminating these high-fat, high-calorie foods from your grocery list. If they're not in the house or in your desk, you won't be tempted. Don't even look at the dessert list at a restaurant. Simply imagining yourself eating a delicious crème brûlée can trigger an intense craving.

One study showed that lack of sleep can lead to eating an extra 900 calories a day.

## Get some shuteye

Research has proven that adults who get 7 to 9 hours of sleep a night eat less during the day and are much less likely to be overweight. For one, when you're sleep-deprived the body produces more of the hormone that causes hunger. Being exhausted also means less willpower to resist the temptation of fatty and sugary foods.

One study showed that lack of sleep can lead to eating an extra 900 calories a day. Wow! Consider that cutting those 900 calories a day for a year would mean a weight loss of more than 90 pounds! To lose weight, you need to give your body the rest it needs. Try going to bed earlier and establishing a routine at night that is calming and gets you ready for deep sleep. For instance, activities like surfing the web or watching TV can disrupt your ability to fall and stay asleep, so try reading for 30 minutes or taking a relaxing bath.

**Trim Up to 200 Calories!**
**Pass:** Croutons
**Swap:** Pita instead of French bread on a sandwich

## Back away from the TV

The National Weight Control Registry (NWCR) is an organization that studies the behavioral and psychological factors that contribute to weight loss and its maintenance. The NWCR tracks more than 5,000 individuals over the age of 18 who have maintained at least a 30-pound weight loss for a year or longer (although the average registry member has lost an average of 66 pounds and kept it off for 5.5 years), and found that there are a few common threads among members. About 80 percent of members report eating breakfast daily and, naturally, almost all members report continuing to maintain a low-calorie, low-fat diet and engaging in high levels of activity. Additionally, 62 percent say they watch less than 10 hours of TV per week. By contrast, the average American watched 38 hours a week, almost 4 times that much. That's nearly as many hours as a full-time job!

Obviously, if you're spending numerous hours a day in front of the TV, you're not exercising. In addition, vegging out leads to overeating of unhealthy foods, out of boredom or for comfort. Who ever curled up on the couch with a salad? As National Weight Control Registry members prove, getting off the couch and away from the TV aids in real weight loss. You'll eat less, and the hours you were spending watching a *Seinfeld* marathon can now be spent hitting the gym, going for a walk with a friend, or otherwise being active outdoors.

## Drink little to no alcohol

Alcohol makes losing weight much tougher. For one, when you drink alcohol, your body processes it first, before fat, protein, or carbs. Thus, alcohol slows down the fat-burning process. Also, a serving of alcohol contains at least 100 calories, and that number can skyrocket if you use sugary mixers. If you take in 100 calories from alcohol, you'll have to find another place to cut it, either with extra exercise or eating less at another meal. That can be very difficult since you're already going to be on a calorie-restricted diet.

Since the goal of this weight-loss plan is to find fast and easy places to cut hundreds of calories, drinking alcohol is

Studies have shown as much as a 20 percent increase in calories consumed at a meal when alcohol was served beforehand.

counterproductive. Plus, it's never smart or healthy to replace nutritious food with alcohol, which offers virtually no nutrients. Also, liquids don't satisfy you or fill you up. In fact, alcohol does quite the opposite. Research has shown that alcohol not only decreases willpower, it may also stimulate the appetite — specifically cravings for fatty and salty foods. Studies have shown as much as a 20 percent increase in calories consumed at a meal when alcohol was served beforehand. So, while it's tough to say no alcohol at all for several weeks, the argument against it is very strong. Most dietitians believe there is no place for alcohol in a reduced-calorie diet.

# Chapter 02

"If you do not change direction, you
may end up where you are heading."

~ Lao Tzu

# Make the Most of Your Metabolism

**We often hear about metabolism** and its importance in helping us lose weight. But what exactly is metabolism, and how can you make yours work harder for you?

Metabolism is a series of chemical reactions that convert the food we eat into energy. This energy powers everything we do, from thinking to moving, healing, growing, and even aging. When you eat, you take in energy in the form of sugars (carbohydrates), proteins, and fats. But the body's cells cannot use energy in this form. So the body must break down these substances so the energy can be distributed to and used by the body's cells. Molecules in the digestive system called enzymes break down each substance differently: proteins are broken down into amino acids, fats are broken down into fatty acids, and carbohydrates are broken down into simple sugars, such as glucose. The process of breaking these substances down and using them for energy is metabolism.

Metabolism is a complicated chemical sequence, so it is easier to think of it in its most basic sense — metabolism is a process that influences how easily you can gain and lose weight, or how easily you store or burn calories. The number of calories you are able to burn in a day depends on how high or low your metabolism is. Earlier in this book, you calculated your basal metabolic rate, or BMR. This is the rate at which your body burns calories while at rest. Everyone has a different BMR, which is largely inherited. You have probably heard friends lament, "Oh, I have the slowest metabolism in the world," or "Have you seen how much so-and-so eats? She must have a super-fast metabolism." However, genetics don't determine everything when it comes to how quickly or slowly your body burns calories. You can actually change your BMR by engaging in certain activities and eating certain foods. For example, regular exercise can increase your body's BMR. Muscle burns 3 times as many calories as fat — about 6 calories per pound for muscle and only 2 calories per pound for fat. Therefore, every extra pound of muscle you put on burns 30 to 50 extra calories per day. Finally, your eating habits — the times at which you eat and your intake of protein or other metabolism-friendly foods — can also increase your BMR.

If you're trying to subsist on carrots, lettuce, and chicken soup, you'll be too exhausted to do much of anything but sit on the couch.

Don't settle for a slow metabolism or use it as an excuse for why you can't lose weight. This chapter gives you all the tips and tricks for super-charging your metabolism, starting from the moment you wake up in the morning.

## Eat breakfast

It's called "the most important meal of the day" for a reason, and eating breakfast is essential for weight loss. Your body is deprived of food during the night — you are literally taking a "break" to "fast." Consider that if you ate dinner the night before at 7 p.m., and you go all the way to lunch without eating, you'll have fasted for 17 hours or more! Your blood sugar will be extremely low. Plus, when your body doesn't receive sufficient nutrients post-fast, it will function less efficiently. Eating a balanced breakfast jump-starts your metabolism, helps you eat a normal portion at lunch, and provides blood-sugar stability that means more energy, brainpower, and focus for your day. And no, a cup of coffee isn't breakfast. Whole grains, oats, peanut butter, fruit, low-fat yogurt, and eggs are all good ways to start your day. They get your metabolism kicking and prevent overeating throughout the day.

### Never skip meals

Dieters make the mistake of believing that skipping meals will help them cut calories and lose weight. But when you skip a meal your system goes into starvation mode. Your metabolism slows down to conserve energy and your body prepares to store fat during your next meal. Additionally, going too many hours between meals means you'll be so hungry, the next time you eat you'll consume far too much. Don't confuse your body by skipping meals; instead, eat small portions throughout the day. Try having 3 small meals and 2 or 3 healthy snacks throughout your day. This keeps your metabolism revved and working continuously, and avoids blood sugar surges and crashes.

## Eat small meals throughout the day

Increase your total calorie-burning capacity by having small, portion-controlled meals throughout the day. The act of eating helps increase your metabolism. The process of absorbing food requires energy. You burn calories with every meal as your body digests food. Keep your metabolism doing its job by spreading out large meals into smaller ones consumed throughout the day. You will end up burning more calories while still eating the same amount of food.

## Eat enough!

Ensure that you are eating enough to keep your metabolism active. Many people mistakenly believe that if they reduce their caloric intake to a very low amount, such as 1,000 calories a day, they'll be able to lose weight more quickly. However, your body and organs, such as the heart, kidneys, and liver, need a certain amount of calories simply to function, much less to get you through a day at work, playing with your kids, and exercising. If you're trying to subsist on carrots, lettuce, and chicken soup, you'll be too exhausted to do much of anything but sit on the couch, and you'll never lose real weight. Find a healthy balance that lets you lose weight but provides enough energy as well.

### Did You Know?

While you may have inherited your metabolism from Mom and Dad, it doesn't mean you can't do something to give a slower metabolism a big boost. Increasing your muscle mass; eating high-protein, low-fat, low-calorie meals and snacks throughout the day; never skipping meals; and being physically active all speed it up naturally!

## Never go too long without eating

Waiting too long between meals can slow down the rate at which your body burns fat, as well as cause blood sugar dips that lead to overeating and feeling sluggish. Instead, try eating every 3 or 4 hours and choose nutritious foods — light cheese and whole grain crackers, small salads, hummus and vegetables, peanut butter on whole wheat toast, baked fish and chicken — and you won't overindulge at any one meal. Keep healthy snacks handy for those days when you're away from your office or house and won't have time to fix something. You never want to go more than 4 hours without putting energizing food in your system.

## Drink coffee and green tea

Coffee can be a helpful diet tool as it suppresses hunger and kick-starts the metabolism. Research shows that green tea can actually help you burn fat and increase your metabolism. Green tea contains very special compounds called catechin polyphenols. These antioxidants help you drop pounds by increasing fat oxidation and thermogenesis, the process where your body temperature increases as a result of burning fat. Green tea can also prevent the storage of excess sugar and fat in the body. Another antioxidant, epigallocatechin gallate (EGCG), has been proven effective at regulating glucose levels which may help reduce your appetite. Drinking 5 cups of green tea may burn 70 to 80 extra calories a day.

Drinking 5 cups of green tea may burn 70 to 80 extra calories a day.

## Stay hydrated!

Maintaining hydration is crucial for weight loss. Water keeps your metabolism working hard, maintains digestion, improves muscle tone, and makes your stomach feel full. Try having a tall glass of water shortly before every meal. How much should you drink? You need to drink at least eight 8-ounce glasses a day. That's the minimum! Men should really strive for 120 ounces of water and women should try to get 90 ounces. If you think about it, it's really not a lot. Buy a regular 750 ml aluminum water bottle (available at any store, from Target to Starbucks to your local gym), fill it up 3 times, and you've already had more than 8 glasses. No matter what your ideal water consumption is, remember to increase water intake in conditions such as high heat, high altitude, low humidity, or high activity level. Water is necessary in order for your metabolism to work properly, so being hydrated helps your body turn food into the energy you need for work, family, and exercise.

### Eat spicy foods

Some research suggests that spicy foods, primarily red pepper, cayenne, and chili pepper, may help raise your metabolism. These foods may increase your calorie burning capacity for up to 2 to 3 hours after eating. The heat generated from capsaicin can increase your body temperature and temporarily raise your metabolic rate by around 8 percent. While studies need to prove whether or not this rate has a profound effect on weight loss, eating spicy foods may also help you lose weight by increasing feelings of satisfaction. The additional water needed to quench the heat from foods may also aid in feeling full when eating a spicy meal.

Men should strive for 120 ounces of water and women should try to get 90 ounces. Increase your intake in high heat, high altitude, low humidity, or high activity level.

### Add lean protein to your diet

Proteins are building blocks for your body. Unlike fat and carbohydrates, which are primarily sources of energy, proteins play an important role in the function and repair of body tissues. Proteins help build muscles and can increase your metabolic rate. It takes more energy for your body to break down protein than it does carbohydrates or fat because of the increased "thermic" effect of digesting protein. In all, the energy it takes just to digest and absorb protein accounts for approximately 25 percent of the total calories protein contains. Ground turkey, skinless white meat poultry, as well as egg whites, fish, and legumes, are great sources of lean protein.

## Eat "negative calorie" foods

Nutrient-rich, fiber-dense foods burn more calories than they contain. Even though fruits and vegetables have calories, they are referred to as "negative calorie" foods. Negative calorie foods usually contain high amounts of nutrients and fiber, and the high fiber content requires more energy to digest than the amount of calories in the food itself. Some negative calorie foods  include asparagus, berries, broccoli, cucumbers, lettuce, grapefruit, oranges, melons, peaches, and plums.

The energy it takes to just digest and absorb protein accounts for approximately 25 percent of the total calories protein contains.

# Chapter

# 03

"When you come to the end of your rope, tie a knot and hang on."

~ Franklin D. Roosevelt

# Plan Ahead for Weight Loss

Your life is packed with commitments that take time and energy, and this also makes it difficult to lose weight. If you are heading to an appointment around meal time, you will probably grab something prepackaged or from the drive-thru, rather than making something fresh and healthy. After a long workday, having pizza and breadsticks delivered to your house sounds much more appealing than cooking a nutritious meal. Or, you might skip out on going to the gym when a friend calls and wants to meet for dinner and drinks. Indeed, work, school, errands, family, friends, and other daily tasks constantly threaten to derail us from working out and eating right. Unless you specifically plan to build healthy habits into your daily life, the best-laid intentions will fall by the wayside. As long ago as 400 B.C., Chinese philosopher Confucius wrote, "When it is obvious that the goals cannot be reached, don't adjust the goals, adjust the action steps." The way you have been living, sacrificing your weight and health in favor of other commitments, is not working. It is critical for the success of this diet program that you don't leave healthy eating to chance. Develop a game plan for how to avoid pitfalls and stick to your healthy habits.

## Stay Motivated!

"Forewarned, forearmed; to be prepared
is half the victory."
~ Miguel de Cervantes Saavedra

Planning ahead, in spite of a busy or stressful schedule, can make all the difference between losing and not losing weight. Determine ahead of time what you will eat at each meal. Build a repertoire of healthy recipes and stock basic ingredients so you'll never be left wondering what to eat. Be prepared with healthy snacks. Make a mental list of the fast food items you can eat without blowing your calorie count. Treat plans to exercise as appointments that cannot be rescheduled.

Burning or saving an extra 500 to 1,000 calories a day will be a challenge already, so you need to properly prepare to make the best food and fitness choices you can. Use the following principles to create a successful game plan for cooking, dining out, creating a calorie budget, and more.

## Make a list of all the healthy foods you enjoy

Facing the reality that you'll need to create a calorie deficit each day for the next few weeks can be overwhelming and daunting. You may feel like there is nothing you can eat when you are trying to lose weight. Make grocery shopping and planning meals easier by writing a complete list of the healthy foods you enjoy. Once you write down all the foods you love that you can still include in your reduced-calorie diet, your options will seem a lot broader and more appealing. Consider the recommended low-fat and low-calorie dairy products, cereal, meat and seafood, soup and canned goods, frozen meals, salad dressings, prepackaged snacks, beverages, treats, and more from the tear-out shopping list in the beginning of this book, and write down your own favorites.

## Plan your meals for the entire week

Don't wait until Monday evening when your stomach is growling to try and decide what to cook for dinner. Use your weekend to plan your menu for the following week. If you plan ahead on Saturday or Sunday, you are already in the mind-set to eat smart and lose weight. Also, you will be less likely to use the weekend as an excuse to overindulge. Take a look at your schedule for the week and decide on a variety of tasty and healthy meals, based on the amount of time you'll have to cook. Then, head to the store to purchase all the ingredients to prepare those meals. Make yourself a quick, healthy lunch option each morning before work — think salads with grilled chicken or salmon, or soup and half a turkey sandwich with veggies. Preparing for the week ahead and making your own meals can save hundreds of calories per meal.

> Unless you specifically plan to build healthy habits into your daily life, the best-laid intentions will fall by the wayside.

### Know your "calorie budget" for each meal

Practice planning ahead by budgeting your calories at each meal. By writing everything you eat or drink in your journal in the back of this book, you will know how many calories you have saved and how many you have to spend on each meal to reach your intake goals. Consider any starters (soup or salad, perhaps), your main course, sides, and beverages. For example, have water: zero calories. Cross "beverages" off your list. Have a small side salad to start. Calories: 150. Have a 250-calorie turkey sandwich, hold the mayo, and you're at 400 calories. Now let's say you had budgeted 500 calories for this meal. You could spend that last 100 calories on a cookie, which provides a few moments of enjoyment, or you could save those last 100 calories. If you make this same choice every day at every meal, you will see the difference on the scale and in the mirror at the end of the week — guaranteed.

## Have a game plan for dining out

A recent study showed that people consume 50 percent more calories, fat, and sodium when they eat out. But just because you're trying to lose weight quickly, doesn't mean you have to pass on dinner with friends — you just need to plan ahead so you don't overeat. According to Purdue University research, eating a pre-meal snack of a handful of peanuts about an hour before dinner will lead you to eat less total calories and fat during your main meal. Also, a broth-based soup or small side salad are good pre-meal choices. To eat less, anticipate what you're going to order, so your eyes don't get bigger than your stomach when you're sitting at the table with all your friends. Almost all restaurant menus are online now, and many also provide nutritional facts, so check ahead of time and decide what you're going to have. Consider ordering an appetizer, such as steamed mussels or a Caprese salad as your meal. Restaurants are notorious for doubling and even tripling portion sizes, so truly, an appetizer or half-portion is probably all the food you need anyway.

### Did You Know?

Research estimates that soft drinks make up between 5.5 and 7 percent of the calories in an American diet! If you haven't already, give up full-sugar soda immediately. However, simply drinking diet soda isn't enough of a weight-loss game plan. Be sure you're not ordering the fried chicken bucket just because you're enjoying a zero-calorie soda.

### Start a recipe folder

When you're trying to decide what to cook, you need an array of healthy options right at your fingertips or you'll be tempted to call for take-out or pick up greasy fast food. Start keeping a recipe folder. Go online and print out healthy recipes from sites like CookingLight.com or EatingWell.com. Or buy magazines like *Real Simple* that offer fast, healthy recipes with complete calorie and fat information, and fill your folder with tear-outs. Better still, contact friends and family who are in good shape and ask for their healthy, tried-and-true recipes. You could even start a healthy-recipe email chain that lots of people you know will benefit from.

## Make a shopping list and stick to it

Focus on shopping for only the items you need to lose weight and stick to the list you made earlier in this chapter. Grocery stores stock the most tempting foods at eye level and in the center aisles. It's easy to get sidetracked if you let your eyes wander. It's also hard to resist a good bargain. Sale items can be difficult to pass up, so avoid the "end caps" of store aisles, which offer low prices on processed items that have a high profit margin, like donuts, sugary cereal, soda, chips and dip, and other unhealthy foods. You will be less susceptible to bright packaging, enticing deals, and other impulse items if you put on grocery shopping blinders and stick to your list.

After a meal, you could spend your last 100 calories on a cookie, which provides a few moments of enjoyment, or you could save those last 100 calories. Save them and you will see the difference on the scale at the end of the week — guaranteed.

## Don't grocery shop when you're hungry

Stores use merchandising tricks such as smell, product placement, overall store layout, and sale items to get you to buy more. These ploys encourage you to shop longer and spend more money. You may end up buying more food than you need, especially if you are hungry. Stop by the grocery store after a meal when you won't be as likely to stray from your shopping list. Or drink a large glass of water. The feeling of fullness will Make it easier to resist food. Another tip is to chew on a piece of peppermint gum while you shop. You will be less likely to try free samples.

## Plan ahead for travel

If you travel often and will be spending a lot of time in airports and on planes in the next few weeks, you must have a strategy that enables you to still lose weight. In-flight snacks are typically chips and crackers, with 200 or more empty calories in each tiny package. Airport food is even worse — pre-made sandwiches, personal pizzas, burritos, and barbecue are common layover fare, so you're looking at up to 800 calories. Ward off extra calories by packing portable, healthy snacks in your carry-on when you are faced with layovers, long flights, or possible delays. Raw, pre-cut veggies, an apple, dried fruits and nuts, and whole wheat crackers with natural peanut butter are easy-to-pack snacks. Or make a sandwich (hold the mayo) that you wrap in tin foil and eat mid-flight. Other travelers will be jealous of your healthy, tasty meal!

## Outsmart the minibar

A weary traveler can easily be tempted by the hotel minibar and its salty and sweet snacks that are just an arm's length away. Practice this celebrity trick and save hundreds of calories by calling your hotel ahead of time and asking that the minibar be locked up or emptied all together. It's too easy to give into temptation when you're on-the-go, so plan ahead for an out-of-town stay. Instead, bring healthy snacks with you or stop by a grocery store to stock up on smart options to keep in your room.

## Keep meal replacement options in your car or desk

There are times when a fresh, home-cooked meal isn't an option, so have some meal replacement bars and shakes on hand. While they aren't a long-term meal substitute, they are certainly the better choice when you need nutrition in a hurry and your other choice is the drive-thru or vending machine. Stick to drinks and bars that provide a balanced 40/30/30 or 40/40/20 ratio of carbohydrates, fats, and proteins. Steer clear of bars with too many simple sugars, which add empty carbs, and don't satiate you over an extended time period. Instead, look for a bar with more fiber, which will make you feel full longer. And stay away from anything that contains partially hydrogenated oils, which are a source of heart-clogging trans fats.

Don't wait until Monday evening when your stomach is growling to try and decide what to cook for dinner. Use your weekend to plan your menu for the following week.

## Cook and freeze meals for later

While fresh is always better than frozen, many busy people enjoy the fact that frozen meals save them time. If you like the efficiency and convenience of frozen diet meals, try taking one evening or weekend afternoon to make a large batch of fresh food that can be divided into servings, frozen, and reheated later. Soup, chili, and vegetarian lasagna are just a few great options that can be made in healthy ways. Store each portion in an airtight container, freeze, and enjoy for up to three months. Having a frozen pre-portioned meal on hand at all times means you won't be tempted to go for fast food when you're short on time.

# Chapter

# 04

"Live to the point of tears."

~ Albert Camus

# Curb Your Appetite

**Our need for food is first and foremost a biological need.** Our body needs calories, fat, nutrients, vitamins, carbohydrates, water, and proteins to carry out complex biochemical reactions that allow us to grow, heal, and function. But of course, if eating were primarily about giving our bodies the energy they need to function, we would simply take a pill or gel that contained our daily nutritional values and call it a day. In reality, eating is a social activity often dictated by our desires for certain kinds of food.

This love of food, or what we call "appetite," however, causes us to eat when we are not hungry, to overeat because we like how a food tastes, to crave foods that are bad for us, and to substitute eating for other activities when we are bored or restless. Our love of eating causes us to forget the primary biological reasons we are supposed to eat. This, combined with technological advances in food preparation and preservation as well as a higher standard of living, provides us with a dizzying array of choices through which to satisfy our hungry stomachs.

Controlling your appetite is one of the most important parts of losing weight in a short amount of time. The best way to curb your appetite is to continually remind yourself that while eating is pleasurable, you should do so primarily because you have a physical need to eat. Food is fuel for your day, for exercise, for mental focus, and for your well-being.

The tips and secrets you learn in this chapter will help you determine what causes you to eat when you're not hungry, restrict your desire for food when your body does not really need it, stave off cravings for high-calorie foods, and eat less overall to lose weight.

## Ask yourself, "What type of hunger is this?"

One key to losing weight is to identify your hunger and stop mindless snacking and eating. People may eat when they're not hungry or they overeat when they are extremely hungry and have low blood sugar. Sometimes people eat more in a social setting, surrounded by friends. Other times, they eat more sitting home alone, out of loneliness or boredom. One specific food may even trigger overeating. Since you cannot avoid food, you need to identify your hunger and find a way to address that need in the right way. Figure out if you are experiencing true physical hunger, low blood sugar hunger, cravings, comfort eating, or social hunger. Once you are honest with yourself about why you're eating, you can put down the chips and wait until you're experiencing true physical hunger to eat a full, healthy meal.

> Indulging in the bad foods you crave forms neuron connections in the brain. When these pathways get constantly activated and reinforced, you end up thinking about and craving those foods all the time.

## Know what foods trigger your appetite

Identify the foods that send your appetite out of control. These are foods that you find yourself compulsively overeating after one bite. Common trigger foods usually combine sugar and fat, or fat and salt. Binges are linked to the food itself; for example, if donuts are one of your trigger foods, a single bite can result in you eating 3 donuts, regardless of your hunger, situation, or emotional state. Until you are able to stop these impulses, you should avoid your trigger foods completely. Avoid even walking past the bakery section at the grocery store. Don't have a box of Girl Scout cookies at home if you know you won't stop with just one cookie. For now, skip the office happy hour if you know you'll be tempted to binge on salty bar food.

## Recognize that seeing foods you crave makes you want them more

Your sense of sight is a key factor in controlling your appetite and losing weight. Research has shown that seeing and indulging in the bad foods you crave over and over forms neuron connections in the brain. When these pathways get constantly activated and reinforced, you end up thinking about and craving those foods all the time. When a person sees a food he or she likes, the brain becomes very active; on the flip side, brain waves show less activity when people look at foods they don't particularly like. Even a photo of a tasty dish can increase your appetite. Don't linger over menus with large images of high-calorie meals and don't even look over at the dessert tray. Don't let your gaze wander to other diners' plates when eating out. Simply recognizing that sight has a significant impact on your appetite will help you fight the temptation to eat when you are not hungry.

## Steer clear of refined carbohydrates

Refined carbs are items made with sugars and white flour, such as white pasta, rice, bagels, donuts, and muffins. Ever notice how your morning bagel actually makes you feel hungrier after you eat it? That's because the body processes refined carbs so quickly that your blood sugar surges and drops. When blood sugar levels drop, the body feels hungry. So, you've not only eaten a 450-calorie bagel with cream cheese, you're ready to eat again mid-morning. Stick to complex carbohydrates that are low in fat and provide healthy protein, such as oatmeal, whole grain rice, yams, beans, and more. These foods slow the digestion process and the release of sugar into the bloodstream to keep levels stable and hunger at bay.

### Did You Know?

You may have heard that red wine is high in healthy antioxidants; however, don't use that as an excuse for drinking alcohol and derailing your weight loss. Red wine contains 100 calories a glass or more, and alcohol is known to stoke the appetite. To benefit from antioxidants, try drinking green or black tea instead.

### Alcohol may make you hungrier

A night of dinner and drinks may sound like a good time, but it's wreaking havoc on your weight loss. The first issue is that liquids don't satisfy you or fill you up. In fact, research has shown that alcohol not only decreases willpower, it whets the appetite and increases cravings for high-sodium, high-fat foods (consider traditional "bar food," like onion rings, burgers, nachos, and hot wings). There can be as much as a 20 percent increase in calories consumed at a meal when alcohol was served beforehand. And with the calories from the alcohol added in, there is a 33 percent total increase in calories. Secondly, after a night of imbibing, the alcohol is what the body breaks down first, before other nutrients, slowing the fat-burning process. The bottom line is, don't drink and eat and you'll save hundreds of calories.

## Slow down!

You eat quickly because of a hectic schedule, because you're on-the-go, or simply because you're a fast eater. However, studies show that people who eat quickly consistently overeat and tend to be more overweight than people who eat slowly. When you eat, your body releases hormones that indicate fullness and tell your brain that you are satisfied. It takes up to 20 minutes for this process to take be complete. During this time, it is very easy to stuff yourself with much more food than you really need if you're eating quickly. Use smaller utensils, take smaller bites, chew your food thoroughly, take a drink of water, and put your utensils down between bites. Try eating half of what's on your plate, wait 10 minutes, then have a few more bites if you're still hungry.

A recent study showed that people consume 50 percent more calories, fat, and sodium when they eat out. Plan ahead so you don't overeat.

## Go minty after meals

Studies have shown that mint flavor and smell may suppress appetite for a short period of time, so brush your teeth or chew a piece of mint gum after meals. The majority of what your brain perceives as taste is actually smell, so if you saturate your sense of smell with a strong odor, like mint, the smell of food will be less appealing and you're less likely to eat more than you need. In one study from Wheeling Jesuit University, 40 people sniffed peppermint every 2 hours for 5 days, then sniffed a placebo for the next 5 days. During the week they smelled the peppermint, they consumed 1,800 fewer calories. Also, if you are susceptible to nighttime snacking, brush your teeth early so you won't be tempted to snack after dinner. If you can, keep a travel-size toothbrush and toothpaste set with you in your car and at work.

## Don't go cold turkey with cravings

Don't make your favorite foods off-limits, because you will immediately crave what you deny yourself. And succumbing to cravings leads to overeating. When you eat sweet, salty or high-calorie foods, your brain releases dopamine and other pleasure chemicals. When you deprive yourself of these foods, your body shifts into hedonism mode, demanding what makes it feel good. In addition, people have a tendency to want what they can't have, what is "forbidden." When you go cold turkey from your favorite foods, you dwell on thoughts of those more, until you give in to your craving and you binge.

Instead, treat yourself in a smart way. Eat pre-portioned amounts of the treats you crave, such as the 100-calorie packs of cookies, crackers, and chips sold at all grocery stores. Everything from Reese's Peanut Butter Cups to Pringles now come in 100-calorie snack sizes. Allow yourself just one of these packages when the craving for something sweet or salty feels truly overwhelming.

Or practice the 85/15 rule that many food-lovers swear by: 85 percent of the time you adhere to your reduced-calorie meal plan, and the other 15 percent you enjoy foods that are purely for pleasure. This amounts to about 2 cheat items per week. For instance, enjoying gooey mac 'n' cheese with your grilled chicken at one meal can help you stay on track through-out the week.

## Be the last person to start eating when dining out

People eat between 40 and 70 percent more food when eating in big groups. We tend to adopt the eating behaviors of the majority, no matter how unhealthy they may be. Be the last to start eating in groups in order to lose weight and keep calories down. Also, recognize that social interactions within groups of people tend to lengthen meal times. Longer meal times increase the likelihood that you will eat more. Don't feel the need to keep up with the table and match each bite of other people's food with your own.

The majority of what your brain perceives as taste is actually smell, so if you saturate your sense of smell with a strong odor, like mint, the smell of food will be less appealing.

## Mix up your routine

Altering your routine can help you avoid the triggers and temptations that cause hunger and overeating. If you typically meet a friend for drinks and appetizers after work on Fridays, this may be a routine that has to change. Interestingly enough, the sights and smells of these familiar places may be triggering your compulsion to eat, not the foods themselves. Meet your friend for coffee one morning instead and order a flavored coffee without milk for a zero-calorie drink. Or, if driving past your neighborhood taco shop every day makes your stomach grumble thinking about mega-calorie burritos, take a different route. You can easily save 500 or more calories just by curbing that craving.

# Chapter 05

"Always bear in mind that your own resolution to succeed is more important than any other."

~ Abraham Lincoln

# Practice Portion Control

**A few years ago, the North American Association** for the Study of Obesity performed a fascinating study on portion control and soup. Some of the 54 participants were given a regular bowl containing a regular portion of soup, and were asked to eat as much of it as they liked. Other participants, however, were given a self-refilling bowl of soup. Soup was automatically piped into the bottom of the bowl as the participants were eating, making it impossible for them to ever reach the bottom. Participants were not told that extra soup was being added to their portion, and the soup was piped in so slowly it was impossible for them to tell that soup was being added as they were eating it.

Researchers found that participants who ate from the self-refilling bowl ate a whopping 73 percent more than participants who ate from a normal bowl. Perhaps more astonishing was the fact that those who ate from the self-refilling bowls did not report feeling any more full than those who ate from the regular bowls. Furthermore, the study found that a person's weight did not affect whether they were likely to keep eating from the self-refilling bowls. Participants eating from the self-refilling bowls included overweight, normal weight, and underweight participants. Across the board, everyone ate more, no matter what their weight or mood.

This study proved what most people have already come to realize: the size of your portion determines how much you will eat, regardless of how hungry you are.

Another interesting study of the factors that lead to over-consumption, published in the *Journal of Consumer Research* in 2008, found that a concept called "extremeness aversion" also contributes to bad portion control, overeating and obesity. Extremeness aversion is the tendency for individuals to avoid the smallest and largest sizes and order the middle size — no matter how large. According to Kathryn M. Sharpe, Richard Staelin, and Joel Huber, the authors of the study, this concept has gradually led retailers to offer larger and larger portions. You may have noticed that businesses like movie theaters and fast food restaurants have begun to inflate the sizes of highly caloric items like popcorn, fries and soft drinks. The study showed that if a fast food restaurant originally offered 21-ounce, 16-ounce and 12-ounce options for soft drinks, most consumers would rule out the large and small sizes and choose the middle size, 16 ounces. However, when the restaurant eliminated the 12-ounce drink, consumers would choose the 21-ounce drink because the 16-ounce size they preferred earlier was now the smallest, or the extreme, making it less desirable.

Additionally, studies have proven that people are terribly inaccurate when it comes to eyeballing correct portions. A study referenced in the *Journal* of *Marketing Research* showed that consumers' perceptions of serving size are highly unreliable and can unknowingly vary as much as 20 percent. Another study showed that consumers vastly underestimate the caloric content of the foods they eat. In a recent study, researchers asked consumers to estimate the number of calories in different fast food meals. Most participants estimated 700 to 800 calories for these meals — about half of the actual amount.

Portion control is three-fold: being aware and anticipating situations in which you may be served large portions, eating smaller portions, and feeling satiated by smaller portions. While this may not be easy at first, you will quickly learn that you can be perfectly happy with much less food than you have been eating. And it should be fairly easy to recognize the  environments in which you are likely to overeat. For example, certain restaurants are well-known for serving outlandish portions — 2 and 3 times the amount you need to eat. Or you may be aware that visiting family means large meals with lots of food. Having a plan going into these situations can help you maintain proper portion control — and self-control.

Use these tips and secrets to keep your portions reasonable and your weight loss on track. Controlling your portion sizes is one of the very best ways to build a substantial calorie deficit each day.

## Know the correct serving size for your favorite foods

Do you know what a single serving is for your favorite foods, such as pasta, chicken, rice, oatmeal, and fruit? The reality of dieting is that you *can* eat most of the foods you love if you exercise portion control. First, that means educating yourself about what one serving of your favorite foods really is!

Keep in mind that certain factors affect food portions, such as the individual's age, gender, and activity level, but according to the USDA, one serving equals:

- 1 slice of whole grain bread
- 1/2 cup of cooked rice or pasta
- 1/2 cup of mashed potatoes
- 3-4 small crackers
- 1 small pancake or waffle
- 2 medium-sized cookies
- 1/2 cup cooked vegetables
- 1/2 cup tomato sauce
- 1 cup lettuce
- 1 small baked potato
- 1 medium apple
- 1/2 grapefruit or mango

- 1/2 cup berries
- ⅓ cup dried fruit or nuts
- 2 tbsps peanut butter
- 1 cup yogurt or milk
- 1 1/2 ounces of cheese
- 1/2 cup dry beans
- 1/2 cup tofu
- 1 chicken breast
- 1 medium pork chop
- 1/4 pound hamburger patty
- 1 tsp butter or margarine

## Learn to eyeball portion sizes

No need for annoying measuring cups or a food scale — a handful here and a scoop there — that looked like a tablespoon, right? Wrong. Research has shown that people can't eyeball portions without some practice. You won't always have a measuring cup on-hand, and who knows what an ounce of something looks like? Create a system in which you associate the size of a familiar object, like a golf ball or your fist, to serving sizes of your favorite foods. You need to learn how to associate common objects with the serving size of foods. After some time, you will be able to recognize correct portions just by how they fill up a plate, bowl, or pan. Here is a list to help you get started, or come up with your own serving-size associations if you like:

- Vegetables or fruit: the size of your fist or a baseball
- Pasta: one handful
- Meat, fish, or poultry: a deck of cards or the size of your palm
- Snacks (chips, pretzels, etc): a cupped handful
- Apple: a baseball
- Potato: a computer mouse
- Bagel: a hockey puck
- Pancake: a CD
- Ice cream: a tennis ball
- Steamed rice: a cupcake wrapper
- Cheese: size of your whole thumb
- Dried fruit or nuts: a golf ball or an egg
- Cereal: a fist
- Dinner roll: a bar of soap
- Peanut butter: a ping pong ball
- Butter or margarine: a postage stamp
- Salad dressing: a ping pong ball

A way to put your frozen dinners to work for weight loss is to save the empty containers, then wash them out and use them as a model for proper portion sizes the next time you cook.

## Create a harmony between carbs, protein & veggies

A simple way to stick with moderate portions is to figure out the proportions of protein, carbohydrates, and vegetables for your meal. Divide your plate into halves. Start out by filling the first half of your plate with non-starchy vegetables, such as a salad, green beans, or grilled tomatoes. Fill a quarter of your plate with protein. Choose from fish, poultry, or lean cuts of beef. The other quarter should be a starchy vegetable or grain like sweet potatoes. Now you can ensure your meal is nutritionally balanced and that you'll feel full and satisfied.

> Create a system in which you associate the size of a familiar object, like a golf ball or your fist, to serving sizes of your favorite foods.

## Order single items rather than combo or meal deals

Fast food restaurants lure customers with combo meals that include a variety of items at a low price. Avoid these marketing ploys no matter how great the value. The amount of calories in a combo meal can contain more than a days worth of calories. For example, a quarter-pound cheeseburger, large fries, and a 21-ounce milkshake has over 1,800 calories. If you have to eat fast food, you can still lose weight by creating your own combo. Places like McDonald's will let you make substitutions, such as apple slices for fries and grilled chicken for breaded and fried chicken. The kids' menu also often includes more reasonable portions.

## Eat from smaller dishware and silverware

One trick that can help control portion size when you're eating at home is using smaller plates, bowls, glasses, and silverware. Think about it: If you're using a large dinner plate, you're more inclined to fill it completely with spaghetti and meatballs — and then eat the whole plate of food. But if you eat with smaller dishware, it gives the impression that there is more food or drink, so your brain will report that you're full and satisfied from a smaller portion. And using smaller spoons and forks means taking smaller bites, eating more slowly, and enjoying your meal longer, giving your body time to feel satiated.

## Stock your freezer with healthy frozen foods

If your freezer is full of healthy frozen entrées as well as frozen meats and vegetables, you won't be tempted to call for take-out or get fast food when you're hungry. Check the reusable grocery list in this book to help you stock up on meals with up to 400 calories and less than 10 grams of fat, as well as items such as frozen peas, broccoli, spinach, berries, boneless and skinless chicken breasts, fish, shrimp, pork loin, ground turkey, and more. On the other hand, items to leave out of your freezer include ice cream, chocolate, alcohol and any other temptations.

## Use frozen diet dinner trays for portion control

An awesome benefit of frozen diet meals is that they are nutritionally balanced, portion-controlled and provide an accurate idea of how much fat, carbs, sodium and calories

Order a "bistro size" or "lunch portion" of salads and entrées. This portion size will leave you happy and full at the majority of restaurants.

you're eating. Another way to put your frozen dinners to work for weight loss is to save a few of the empty containers when you're done eating. Wash them out and use them as a model for proper portion sizes the next time you cook. Frozen diet meals can be an excellent teacher for understanding the right ratios of protein, vegetables. starch, and sauce.

> ### Trim Up to 200 Calories!
> **Pass:** Garlic bread or breadsticks
> **Swap:** Spray salad dressing instead of bottled dressing

## Don't put serving dishes out on the table

Part of losing weight and exercising portion control is feeling satiated from a smaller amount of food than you're used to. It's important to know that sense of satiation is very visual. If you set bowls or pans of food out on the table, you are simply encouraging yourself to take seconds. Serve yourself a reasonable portion size while you're in the kitchen, then put the rest of the food away for leftovers. This way you won't be tempted to take more of anything. Savor and appreciate each bite. After you eat, busy yourself with dishes and cleaning up your cooking space — this gives your brain a chance to register that your body is full, and you won't feel the need to grab another dinner roll or helping of potatoes.

## Take the food out of its container

When you're eating out of a container, there is also a tendency to feel like you haven't eaten enough to satisfy you. If you take the food out of the packaging your brain will register just how much you're really eating. A yogurt may not look like much in its packaging, but you'll discover its contents actually fill a bowl. And how many times have you gotten to the bottom of a 100-calorie snack pack and commented, "There were only four cookies in there!" If you pour them out ahead of time, your brain has a chance to register that you are, in fact, eating a full handful of small cookies, which is a healthy portion for losing weight.

## Order the smallest size meal when dining out

We all know that portion control is much easier when we're eating at home. At home we can regulate how much we put on a plate, whereas at a restaurant, portions are often 2 and even 3 times the size of what we'd serve ourselves. A huge part of losing weight is learning to identify a smart portion when dining out. Always opt for the smallest portion size available.

Many restaurants offer a "bistro size" or "lunch portion" of their salads and entrées. This portion size will leave you happy and full at 99 percent of restaurants. Or order an appetizer version of a full entrée, such as a veggie quesadilla or steamed mussels. When you find yourself wondering, "Will the half salad be enough?" remember that restaurants often inflate portion sizes in order to charge more. Cut calories (and save money) by opting for the smaller portion.

After you eat, busy yourself with dishes and cleaning up your cooking space — this gives your brain a chance to register that your body is full, and you won't feel the need to grab another dinner roll or helping of potatoes.

### Exercise nut portion control!

While studies have shown that people who include nuts in their diets often have lower risk of heart disease, nuts are also very calorie-dense, much of which is from fat. Nuts are only beneficial if they are eaten in careful moderation and do not significantly contribute to your daily calorie count. Unfortunately, because nuts come in large tins and bags, it is just too easy to snack on them by the handful and wreak havoc on your weight loss.

Know that not all nuts are created equal! Good nuts include almonds, walnuts, peanuts and pistachios. Not-so-good nuts, such as macadamias, pecans, and Brazil nuts, are high in fat and calories. Because all nuts are calorie-dense, stick to about an ounce of nuts, which equals 160 to 200 calories.

NutHealth.org lists the following as the number of nuts per serving:

- Almonds: 20-24
- Cashews: 16-18
- Macadamias: 10-12
- Brazil nuts: 6-8
- Hazelnuts: 18-20
- Pecans: 18-20 halves
- Pistachios: 45-47
- Pine nuts: 150-157
- Walnuts: 8-11 halves

Nuts make an easy, crunchy snack, just make sure you always count them out into snack-size baggies. Never try to ration while eating from a jar or bag of nuts — you'll overdo it. And be smart: Pass on anything honey-roasted, candied, oil-roasted, or covered in chocolate or yogurt. Raw, unsalted, unroasted nuts are the ones that will make you feel full and satisfied while keeping your calories down. In the right portions, they can be part of a successful weight-loss plan.

Extremeness aversion is the tendency to avoid the smallest and largest sizes and order the middle size — no matter how large. Be wary of this when you order items like movie theater popcorn and soda at fast food restaurants, and always stick to the smallest size.

### Ask for a doggie bag right away

Another smart dieter's trick is to ask for a doggie bag or to-go container as soon as your entrée touches down on the table. Determine an appropriate portion and set aside the rest for leftovers. When the entire meal stays on your plate, you are constantly tempted to keep eating and eating until your plate is bare. Think about how many times you've thought, *Well, I've eaten two-thirds of this meal already, so I may as well finish the rest.* Store half your meal out of sight and feel content when the plate is empty.

## Split your meal in half

You can cut calories and still enjoy your favorite foods by dividing your meal and only eating half. One way to do this is to split your meal with a friend. Or, if you and your dining companion can't agree, you can substitute the other half of your meal with a broth-based soup, fresh veggies, or a piece of fruit. For instance, instead of 2 slices of pepperoni pizza, replace the second piece of pizza with a garden salad and light dressing. This simple change can save you about 350 calories. Substitute water with lemon or sparkling water, like Perrier, instead of a soda, and you've saved 500 calories right there.

People who include nuts in their diet often have lower risk of heart disease; however, enjoy them in moderation, because nuts are very calorie-dense.

# 06

"Divide each difficulty into as many parts as
is feasible and necessary to resolve it."

~ René Descartes

# No More Mindless Eating!

**With our busy lives and schedules,** so much of eating happens while we multitask or are on-the-go — at desks, in front of the TV, with friends, or in cars. Unfortunately, eating while distracted or while working on something else leads to overeating. Mindless eating is the downfall of many dieters. The hand-to-mouth action of eating can become addictive and, before you know it, you've gone through a large bag of chips or eaten an entire plate of fries that you didn't even order! Losing weight comes from holding yourself accountable — including your guilty pleasures, little indulgences, and bad habits.

You must learn to pay attention while food is around you. One key is, of course, keeping a food diary, which is the single-best way to stay accountable for and aware of what you're eating. Stop functioning on auto-pilot and start paying attention to what you're eating, when you're eating, and where you're eating. Most environments offer cues and clues that may tempt you to eat too much, and you must pay attention to those and get your willpower ready. You probably also harbor several unconscious habits that cause you to snack and eat without even realizing it. These are opportunities to change your behavior and cut hundreds of extra calories from your day!

Because food provides pleasure and comfort for so many people, and because calories sneak up on you in so many places, you must stop mindlessly eating in order to lose weight fast. Wake up! Pay attention! Savor the healthy foods you eat but make eating an experience more about fueling your body than about enjoyment. Truly, the most wonderful feeling will be when you step on the scale at the end of each week and see the weight dropping off!

Just like the old adage, "Don't grocery shop while you're hungry," don't cook while you're starving either. Start making a meal before you're hungry so you don't snack while cooking.

### Keep a food diary!

A hugely important step to eating fewer calories and burning through unwanted pounds is keeping a food diary. Keeping track of what you eat and drink keeps you accountable and aware, and prevents mindless snacking. Luckily, this journal comes equipped with a food and fitness log, but you'll want to keep maintaining one even after you've lost weight. Why? For one, you probably have no idea how many calories or grams of fat are in much of what you eat. Research has shown again and again that people grossly underestimate the number of calories in their food — they are usually off by about 50 percent! Additionally, people tend to have generous and selective memories when it comes to what they have eaten. How many times have you "forgotten" about a half of a muffin, a handful of crackers, or finishing your child's cookie?

A study in the *American Journal of Preventive Medicine* followed 1,700 overweight or obese men and women (the average weight was 212 pounds) who were following an exercise and diet plan. The subjects who did not record what they ate lost 9 pounds. However, those who did keep a food journal lost twice as much weight, or an average of 18 pounds. So keep your food and fitness journal up-to-date and be accountable for every bite and sip!

## Are you a snacking chef?

Are you constantly "taste testing" your chili every few minutes? Do you snack on shredded cheese while you're dicing taco toppings? Does licking the egg beaters after making a dessert date back to a childhood habit? What's the point of preparing a healthy meal for yourself or your family if you're snacking the whole time, adding hundreds of extra calories? Just like the old adage, "Don't grocery shop while you're hungry," don't cook while you're starving either. Start making a meal before you're hungry so the food is ready by the time you're eager to eat. If it's too late and you're already hungry, set aside a small plate of veggies, such as carrots or crunchy cucumber slices, to enjoy while you cook. A spoonful of peanut butter or a few crackers can also hold you over for a while so you aren't tempted to lick the bowl after making banana bread. Start paying attention when you cook and don't let hundreds of needless calories sneak in.

## Beware of drive-by snacking

Food is often presented in a way that makes it seem casual, easy, and friendly: a bowl of M&M's on someone's desk at work; kiosks of samples at Costco; attractive hors d'oeuvres at a party; or a tray of bite-sized tasters at the coffee shop. Without thinking, you grab a handful of candy each time you walk to your cubicle. At a party, you take something off every tray of hors d'oeuvres that comes around. As you chat with friends, "Ooh, I'll try that," becomes, "Sure, I'll have another." Soon you have a pile of cocktail napkins and crumbs in your hand. People often have the misconception that a few bites here and a few bites there are OK — but they add up quickly. You must eliminate drive-by snacking if you're going to cut out the hundreds of calories you need to reach your weight-loss goal. Avoid opportunities for mindless snacking. Don't spend a long time chatting with a coworker who has candy or cookies at his or her desk, but if you must, be mindful of the presence of temptation and don't give in!

## Did You Know?

How many food-related choices do you think you make in a day? When a Cornell University team of researchers posed this question to participants, the average answer was 14. However, when the participants were asked to more closely consider a typical day, it showed that they actually made an average of 226 food decisions a day. One author of the study concluded: "It is not unfair to say we often engage in mindless eating."

## Look out for liquid calories!

Are you drinking your calories? Juice, smoothies, sweetened tea, sports drinks, energy drinks, protein shakes, and alcohol are all packed with calories, sugar, and carbs — just like soda, and sometimes more so. Plus, have you ever looked closely at the labels of your Gatorade, Naked Juice, Arizona Iced Tea or Monster? Most bottled drinks contain more than 1 serving — 2.5 servings per bottle is typical. If you drink the whole bottle, which most people do, you're drinking 200 to 400 calories in just a few gulps. The real problem is that liquids don't fill you up, so you wind up eating on top of what you're drinking. Satiation comes from chewing, thus many times a liquid will be ingested unconsciously in just a few gulps, without helping you feel full, and without any thought of the calories you just consumed. It's easy to forget about 250 calories when they're in liquid form, but cutting out 250 calories can make a big difference in the amount of weight you lose. Drinks are a quick and easy place to cut extra calories to lose more weight.

## Beware of bite-sized

Unfortunately, our brains often trick us into thinking that eating something bite-sized means it's better for us than eating the same food in its full size. But this is only true if you eat just a few bite-sized pieces! And studies have shown that small treats, such as mini-cookies, actually lead people to eat more than they would if the cookies were full-size. If you wouldn't eat a whole cheese Danish, why eat four samples at the coffee shop? You're not doing your waistline any favors, and you're actually doing yourself a double disservice by pretending those calories don't count. Whenever samples of high-calorie treats are nearby, such as pastries at a coffee shop, remind yourself that even small bites add up to hundreds of calories.

## Be the life of the party without overindulging

Always eat consciously. At a party, be wary of the hand-to-mouth motion while you're chatting with friends. You don't need to accept every time a waiter comes by offering hors d'oeuvres. Hors d'oeuvres are always rich and fatty in order to pack lots of flavor in a small bite. Items like filled puff pastries, crab cakes, deviled eggs, bacon-wrapped shrimp, and creamy dips are popular and each has a ton of

Are you drinking your calories? Juice, smoothies, sweetened tea, sports drinks, energy drinks, protein shakes, and alcohol are all packed with calories, sugar, and carbs — just like soda, and sometimes more so.

calories. You could be consuming 100 calories or more per bite! When you attend an event or party, stand away from the entrance to the kitchen so you're not the first guest that servers with hot, fresh trays of hors d'oeuvres see. Also, a great calorie-saving trick for parties is to fill up lighter fare, such as crunchy crudités (raw veggies), shrimp cocktail, or smoked salmon, and allow yourself only one indulgent treat. Eat one bite to be sure it's truly delicious and worth the calories. If it's not, toss the rest away.

A study in the journal, *Obesity*, reported that people consume an average of 236 more calories on Saturdays than on any other day of the week.

## Never eat in front of the TV

More than 66 percent of Americans report that they regularly watch TV while dining at home. Unfortunately, people who watch television while eating tend to overeat without being aware of it. Studies have shown that people can eat almost an entire extra meal's worth of calories on days when they eat in front of the TV. Television distracts you from responding naturally to your body's cues of hunger and fullness. Turning on the TV can trigger the desire to snack even if you are not hungry. You also tend to rely on external cues, such as the end of a show, rather than internal cues to stop eating. Keep the TV off and sit down at the table to savor the flavor, color, and texture of your food. You'll eat hundreds fewer calories than you would zoning out on the couch.

## Keep food far from your bedside

Having food in bed is a habit that dates back to childhood for many people. You may have enjoyed a warm glass of milk in bed in order to have a better night of sleep. Maybe your mother brought you soup when you weren't feeling well. Or perhaps the concept of "breakfast in bed" was seen as an indulgence meant for Dad on Father's Day. Whatever the case may be, know that eating in bed only promotes mindless eating. Bringing a bag of popcorn or a tub of ice cream into bed while you watch a movie or curl up with a book is simply setting the stage for overeating (not to mention making a mess!). Again, practice conscious eating by keeping food in the setting in which it belongs — at the dinner table.

## Look out for overeating cues

Environments that lead to overeating tend to give you cues and clues that too much food is on its way — now you just have to pay attention to them! Family style serving dishes, heaping bread baskets, short and wide drink glasses, carafes of soda or wine, buffet-style presentation, and oversized pasta and salad bowls are simply putting the temptation to grossly overeat in front of you. It's not just restaurants that are the culprit either; take a look around your own home for these items as well. Make your home less conducive to overeating and stay better aware of portion control.

In a portion of the Cornell Food and Brand Lab study "Mindless Eating: The 200 Daily Food Decisions We Overlook," researchers measured the amount eaten by 379 participants, half of whom were served with a particularly large bowl or plate of food. The participants given the extra-large servings ate an average of 31 percent more food than the participants with the normal-sized dinnerware. More interestingly, even when researchers later revealed to those participants that they had been given an extra-large portion, 21 percent denied having eaten more, 75 percent attributed it to other reasons (such as hunger), and only 4 percent attributed it to the environmental cue

> Pay attention to environmental cues and clues that too much food is on its way. Family style serving dishes, carafes of soda or wine, buffet-style presentation, and oversized pasta and salad bowls are simply putting the temptation to grossly overeat in front of you.

of the oversized plate or bowl. Researchers concluded that we are either unaware of how our environment influences eating decisions or we are unwilling to acknowledge it.

Don't be one of the many people who is biased by the size of packaging, presentation, and plating. Look for common cues, and clues and either stay away from environments that offer the temptation to overeat or be so conscious of the temptation that you monitor your intake carefully.

**Trim Up to 300 Calories!**
**Pass:** Cheese slices on sandwiches
**Swap:** Chocolate milk instead of a chocolate milkshake

## Make your own 100-calorie snack packs

Never snack on things like popcorn, nuts, dried fruit, or crackers straight from the bag or package; you'll definitely overdo it. Bags and boxes of snack foods make it difficult to determine a proper portion size. Instead, make your own 100-calorie snack packs so you'll never be without a healthy, low-calorie snack. Put baby carrots, celery sticks, almonds, dried apricots, and whole wheat crackers into small baggies and have them in your purse, desk, backpack, or wherever you'll need them.

TV can trigger the desire to snack, and you tend to rely on external cues, such as the end of a show, rather than internal cues to stop eating. Keep the TV off and sit down at the table to savor your food.

While 100-calorie packs of treats, such as cookies, chips, and candy, are now available, you should only purchase those tempting, sugary or salty snacks if you know you have the willpower to eat just one package. If chocolate chip cookies or potato chips are a trigger food for you, 100-calorie packs are just needless temptation.

## Beware of Saturday diet sabotage

A study in the journal, *Obesity*, reported that people consume an average of 236 more calories on Saturdays than on any other day of the week. Theories on why? For one, your weekends aren't as structured as weekdays, where you have set times for lunch breaks, dinner, etc. Thus, people tend to eat carelessly and at odd times. Also, people tend to the view the weekend as time to relax and take a break from the routine of the workweek, thus, they tend to turn

Hors d'oeuvres are always rich in order to pack flavor in a small bite. Items like filled puff pastries, crab cakes, deviled eggs, bacon-wrapped shrimp, and creamy dips can have 100 calories or more per bite!

their backs on their diets and seriously overeat. However, losing weight quickly requires structure, and not just Monday through Friday. Don't let a lazy Saturday lead you to indulge in a calorie-rich meal. If you want to think of Saturday as a day to take it easy, use it as one of your days off from working out. But that's all the more reason to pass on a fatty meal!

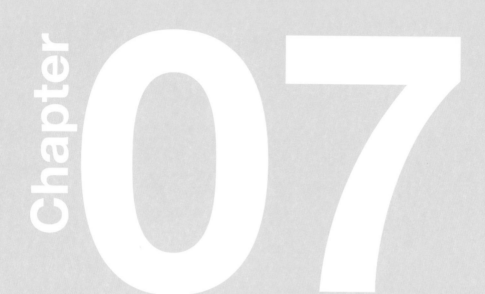

# Chapter 07

"Let us not be content to wait and see what will happen, but give us the determination to make the right things happen."

~ Horace Mann

# No More Emotional Eating

**Ever heard of eating your feelings?** Emotional eating is a huge problem for overweight people and those trying new diets because the very nature of being overweight causes stress, anxiety, sadness, and loneliness — all which contribute to the cycle of emotional eating. Additionally, despite what many people believe, emotional eating is *not* just a female problem. True, most guys aren't crying into a pint of Häagen-Dazs after a breakup, but millions of men still deal with this major weight-loss roadblock on a daily basis.

A study published in the journal, *Obesity*, reported that people who practice emotional eating have a much harder time losing weight, and those who do lose weight are more likely to regain it. The study concluded that, to be truly successful, weight-loss programs needed to teach their clients coping skills to replace emotional eating practices.

Emotional eating is simply a coping strategy. Anything from relationship problems to unemployment to depression to work-related stress can lead to emotional eating. Many times, emotional eating habits are ingrained and reinforced in us over the years, as we get older and responsibilities and stresses increase with adulthood. And, unfortunately, emotional eaters are typically only interested in fatty or sugary snacks that completely derail their diet plans.

As this chapter reveals, positive emotions and people you love may be causing you to emotionally eat as well. You'll learn to recognize the triggers that lead you to overeat out of celebration, or the friends and loved ones who mean well but are actually wreaking havoc on your weight.

This chapter reveals fascinating facts about how eating in a social setting, with your significant other, family members, or coworkers can determine how much and what you eat. You'll also learn about how your gender affects your calorie intake.

In reality, emotional eating revolves around having a very unhealthy relationship with food — using it as a coping mechanism, a comfort, a distraction from your problems, a means to fit in, or a reward. And when emotional eating spirals out of control, it becomes binge eating, the most common form of disordered eating, which affects approximately 2 million Americans, according to the National Institute of Mental Health. Binge eating disorder, like emotional eating, involves uncontrollable, excessive eating, followed by feelings of shame and guilt. The National Institute of

Mental Health estimates that men account for about 40 percent of binge eaters.

Whether you're overeating in a group of friends or pigging out on late night junk food when you're home alone, you need to confront your bad habits and find better ways to cope with emotional changes and disruptions. Because emotional eating habits are some of the most difficult to change (as they often date back decades to childhood), these are also the behaviors that frustrate people and keep them from losing significant weight.

Feeling powerless to food and your weight is a daily struggle. But learning the emotional triggers, people and situations that lead you to make unhealthy choices is the only way to break the nasty cycle of overeating that causes sadness and anxiety (and, in turn, more overeating). Wouldn't you love to feel in control of your eating habits for once in your life? Wouldn't you love to find other, healthy ways to address stress, conflict, personal issues or to celebrate without ruining your weight-loss efforts? Read on to figure out how to eat for nutrition and weight loss rather than feeding your feelings.

> Because emotional eating habits are some of the most difficult to change (as they often date back decades to childhood), these are also the behaviors that frustrate people and keep them from losing significant weight.

## Recognize that emotional eating makes you feel worse

Emotional eating is a horrible cycle because it both stems from and creates feelings of sadness, stress and embarrassment. How many times have you heard someone say: "I eat because I'm sad, and then I'm sad because I'm fat?" People will binge on ice cream or alcohol when they feel sad, and then, in turn, feel much worse after realizing how many empty calories they just ingested. And the more overweight people get, the more they isolate themselves and soothe themselves with food.

As David L. Katz, M.D., a professor of public health and medicine at Yale University School of Medicine, says, "You can't make food the solution to every issue in your life and expect to be thin." Stop burying your thin, happy self under high-calorie meals! Your goal of losing weight quickly can be met with awareness, willpower, and dedication. Once you realize how much better you feel from eating healthy and losing weight, you'll never want to fall into the cycle of emotional eating again.

## Recognize these amazing differences between emotional hunger and physical hunger

You must learn the differences between and recognize the cues of emotional and physical hunger to find ways to deal with cravings and avoid overeating. There are several ways to tell whether what you're experiencing is true, internal hunger or whether your body and mind are responding to external emotions. Emotional hunger comes on suddenly, out of nowhere, and is associated with an event or emotion, such as having a fight with your spouse. Physical hunger is gradual; it comes on slowly and includes physical cues, such as a grumbling stomach, hunger pains, or slight fatigue. Emotional eating is typically for a specific food — chocolate or a cheeseburger — and needs to be satisfied immediately. Real, physical hunger can wait several minutes or even hours and a wide range of foods will satisfy it. Emotional hunger is not really related to fullness, so you may eat very quickly and won't stop eating when you feel full. You may also feel distracted and find that you eat a

> ### Did You Know?
> How common is emotional eating? Emotional eating may be a factor in as much as 75 percent of all overeating, according to the Department of Nutrition Therapy at the Cleveland Clinic.

whole bag of chips or box of cookies without realizing it. Physical hunger, however, responds to fullness, and you will stop eating when you're satisfied. Likewise, you eat consciously and slowly, enjoying your food. Emotional hunger is coupled with feelings of guilt and shame for overeating, whereas physical hunger is not accompanied by negative feelings. With physical hunger, you recognize food as fuel, and eating as a necessary part of your day. Finally, emotional hunger may come on soon after you've already eaten. If you feel a craving coming on an hour or two after your last meal or snack, you can bet it's probably not true, physical hunger. With these differences in mind, you should be able to determine which type of hunger you're experiencing. If it's not physical hunger, focus on putting a stop to the craving instead of indulging it.

> Emotional hunger is coupled with feelings of guilt and shame for overeating, whereas physical hunger is not accompanied by negative feelings. With physical hunger, you recognize food as fuel, and eating as a necessary part of your day.

### Head off emotional eating at the pass

Eating out of emotion is what is a called a "negative coping pattern," meaning that you are simply compounding your problems by being overweight. Awareness means stopping emotional eating before it starts. Figure out which types of bad feelings and situations lead you to eat out of emotion rather than hunger. The five most typical emotions or states that cause overeating are loneliness, boredom, anger, stress, and fatigue. If your hand ends up in the bottom of the Snackwells after a fight with your sister, make a mental note of it. If your first reaction to an extra-stressful day at work is to stop for a cheeseburger and 6-pack of beer on the way home, be aware of that negative coping pattern. Then you will be able to anticipate and stop emotional eating down the road.

## Remove temptation!

It sounds basic, but if you don't have trigger foods around the house, you'll have fewer opportunities to overeat. You know the kinds of snacks and desserts you crave late at night, when you're watching a movie or when you've had a bad day. Now, make a list of the things you can have instead — a 100-calorie serving of popcorn, raw veggies, a low-fat yogurt, or low-sugar cereal.

### Trim Up to 500 Calories!

**Pass:** New England clam chowder

**Swap:** Taco salad instead of a burrito (just don't eat the fried bowl!)

## Find other outlets for celebration or comfort

You got fired, you got a promotion, you broke up with your boyfriend, your team won the Super Bowl — so you eat half a pizza. You tell yourself, "I deserve this." You use food to both celebrate and to help you lick your wounds. But what sense does it make to let circumstances largely out of your control so greatly affect your diet and weight? Why would you want the glow of a new job to be outshined by the guilt you feel for eating a pound of Buffalo wings at your celebratory happy hour? Don't use food as comfort or celebration. Find other ways to give yourself a pat on the back or relieve anger and stress during a trying time. Had a great day? Go shopping and treat yourself to a new pair of shoes. Do something that makes you feel great other than overindulging in food, like getting a massage. Had a crappy day? Need a shoulder to cry on? A burrito isn't going to provide the emotional support you need. Call a friend instead. Or sweat it out at the gym. Exercise is the number one stress reliever. And obviously, when you're exercising you're doing something beneficial for your body, as opposed to indulging in a calorie-packed meal.

## Recognize if a friend or loved one is sabotaging your weight loss

While it is natural to expect that the ones who care for you would want to support you in your efforts to lose weight, many people find that certain friends and family members actually sabotage their weight loss — intentionally and unintentionally. Take a look at the person in question — typically, he or she is also struggling with weight, overeating, and a sedentary lifestyle. Some people feel better about their unhealthy lifestyle choices when you live the same way. Many times, the person you are closest to has long been your partner in crime when it comes to unhealthy eating. He or she will feel isolated and jealous when you start making better food choices and pass on the beer-and-pizza Saturdays that have become your tradition. Explain to this person that losing weight and keeping it off is going to require a complete lifestyle makeover, and you want and need his or her love and support to be successful.

> While it is natural to expect that the ones who care for you would want to support you in your efforts to lose weight, many people find that certain friends and family members actually sabotage their weight loss — intentionally and unintentionally.

## Stop the late night snack attack

Dietitians and nutritionists commonly say that late night eating is their clients' biggest problem that keeps them from losing weight. They eat smartly all day only to fall victim to the midnight munchies. Does that sound like you? Learn to ward of the late night snack attack by determining why you're tempted to eat so late. There is an off-chance that you've restricted your calories so much throughout the day that you're actually hungry before bed. If so, try adding more fiber or protein to your dinner to feel fuller longer.

But truly, late night snacking is just another form of emotional eating. Loneliness, boredom, and stress are three of the most typical emotions that cause eating for reasons other than hunger, especially when you're home late at night. To avoid eating out of the desire for comfort or to relax, look for other things to fulfill this need, such as a bath or exchanging massages with your spouse. If you know you're going to be unwinding at home, find something to do with your hands other than eating, such as drinking a mug of tea. Warm liquids are also said to have a calming and de-stressing effect that helps get ready for a good night of sleep. Or, find an activity that includes both hands so you won't have one hand on your book and the other in a bag of Doritos. Type an email to a friend or knit. Cleaning can also be a good stress reliever that keeps you busy and out of the fridge. Whatever it takes, tell yourself you're done eating for the night after you have a healthy dinner.

> Maintain your willpower when eating with friends! A study showed that when men were at the table, a group of women ate about 450 calories each. By contrast, in an all-female group, the number rose to about 750 calories.

## Don't eat more in the company of others — male or female

A 2009 study in the journal, *Appetite*, reported the effects of eating in social settings on both men and women, and discovered that women who ate in all female groups ate significantly more than if they ate alone, on a date, or in a group that included men. When men were at the table, the women ate about 450 calories each. By contrast, in an all-female group, the number rose to about 750 calories. Interestingly, while men were not affected by the gender of their company, they consumed more than 700 calories per meal regardless, which was higher than all the women in the study.

The bottom line is, social environments lead to poor impulse control and overeating. Surely you've heard the phrase, "Eat, drink, and be merry." If your mind-set is that eating out with friends is an indulgence or treat, you're more likely to indulge in high-calorie food, desserts, and drinks. Both sexes should feel confident enough to say "No thanks" when a dinner companion suggests splitting the fried calamari or cheesecake. Alcohol and coffee drinks also rack up major calories, so order hot tea if everyone is having after-dinner drinks. Or suggest social activities that don't include eating! Do something exercise-related, such as arranging for a group bike ride, hike, or entering a 5k with friends.

The five most typical emotions or states that cause overeating are loneliness, boredom, anger, stress, and fatigue.

### Know the few times when it's OK to give in

Certain holidays and special occasions, such as a birthday, Thanksgiving, family reunion, or New Year's Eve, mean you will want to indulge in a rich dessert, buttery mashed potatoes or a few glasses of champagne — and you have to know that it's OK to do so. Treating yourself, rarely and only when the occasion is particularly meaningful, shows a healthy and well-balanced approach to eating. You're not using to food to celebrate per se, but you're enjoying a special moment with loved ones that includes a dietary indulgence. Just plan ahead. If you know you're going to spend a few hundred calories on these treats, you need to plan throughout the day and week to cut back in other areas.

"Develop success from failures.
Discouragement and failure are two of the
surest stepping stones to success."

~ Dale Carnegie

# Choosing Healthy Alternatives

**Americans tend to run in the other direction** when they hear the word "healthy." Indeed, many people mistakenly believe that foods that are healthy are unsatisfying or taste bad. In a new *Journal of Consumer Research* study, researchers found that when people were asked to taste food described as "healthy," they reported being hungrier afterward than those who ate the same food when it was described as "tasty." In one portion of the study, some students were told they were sampling a new protein, vitamin, and fiber-packed "health bar;" others were told it was a "chocolate bar that is very tasty and yummy with a chocolate-raspberry core." When they were later asked to rate their hunger, those who sampled the "health bar" rated themselves hungrier than those who ate the identical "tasty" bar. In a second portion of the study, participants were given a piece of bread either described as being "low-fat and nutritious" or "tasty, with a thick crust and soft center." After sampling the bread, participants were offered pretzels; those who ate the "healthy" bread ate more pretzels than those who sampled the "tasty" bread. This study showed that not only do people expect healthy food to be unsatisfying, it actually makes them hungrier than if they had eaten nothing at all. In the end, "healthy" foods made subjects eat in excess.

As a nation, we have been somewhat brainwashed to view reduced or low-fat foods as second-class to the original. But in many cases, reduced fat or low-cal foods are indistinguishable from their higher calorie counterparts. Sometimes, the low-fat version is actually tastier! To lose weight fast, you need to change your perception that healthy foods will not satisfy you as much as your favorite dishes. In fact, you will probably find that once you continuously substitute vegetables, fruits, and whole grains for greasy, fried fast food meals, you will start to prefer the fresh, clean taste of lower-calorie foods.

Half of a large grapefruit has 50 calories, 2 grams of fiber, and 11 grams of sugar while 8 fluid ounces of grapefruit juice contains about 100 calories and 22 grams of sugar. When you're craving something sweet and juicy, reach for the real piece of fruit rather than juice.

In order to lose weight, you must make healthy trade-offs. Giving up desserts in favor of fruit, for instance, can help you drop unwanted pounds quickly. Or eating out less and cooking at home more — though eating out may be more fun — saves hundreds of calories at each meal. In weight loss, trade-offs usually mean giving up something you enjoy for something less instantly gratifying but healthier in the long run. Diet trade-offs are worth it because reaching an ideal weight, feeling great and being healthier are the ultimate payoffs.

Nothing will be more motivating than recognizing bad habits, beginning new ones, and seeing the unwanted pounds come off! Mark Twain once joked, "The only way to keep your health is to eat what you don't want, drink what you don't like, and do what you'd rather not." But this doesn't have to be true! Being healthy and slimming down is really all about making smart trade-offs that have real benefits to you.

## Modify recipes with healthy ingredient substitutions

There's no need to toss out your favorite recipes — just find healthy substitutions for the high-calorie ingredients. Your favorite dishes will retain their flavor and save you hundreds of calories. You won't even notice the difference! A favorite diet secret is substituting Greek or other non-fat yogurt for sour cream and mayo. You won't lose any of the creaminess but with zero grams of fat and the multitude of protein, you're making a smart trade-off. Tofu is also good substitute for many ingredients because it is rich in high-quality protein and contains no cholesterol. Try using it in place of cream in sauces. Replace ground beef with lean ground chicken or turkey. If a vegetable recipe calls for butter or margarine, use chicken broth and herbs for flavor without the fat. Replace whole eggs with two egg whites and just a tiny bit of yolk. Use condensed skim milk for whole milk. Replace the sugar in baking recipes with the no-calorie sweetener Splenda.

## Choose the right salad dressings

Salads can, of course, be one of your best weight-loss friends. Frequently eating green salads with raw veggies means your body will be getting crucial nutrients and antioxidants, such as vitamins A, C, and E, folic acid, fiber, lycopene, and beta-carotene. However, to slim down quickly, you need to be consider the dressings you're choosing. A study of 1,000 people by Kraft Foods found that the top choices of salad dressing for women were Ranch, blue cheese, and vinaigrette. Men's top choices were Ranch, blue cheese, French/Catalina, and Thousand Island. Clearly, creamy dressings are the favorites of both men and women. They are also the quickest way to turn your healthy meal into salad sabotage. And beware of vinaigrettes that load up with sugar to achieve better taste.

To save hundreds of calories and dozens of grams of fat, ask for oil and vinegar. A few splashes of balsamic or red wine vinegar are often all you need on a vegetable salad. Even better? Squeeze a fresh lemon over your salad for a zero-calorie dressing. If you can't live without your favorite dressings, many, such as Caesar and raspberry vinaigrette, come in a spray bottle version with only 1 calorie per spray (10 sprays are enough for a 1-cup salad). Don't turn your healthy salad into a 1,000-calorie nightmare; choose the right dressings.

## Cook veggies the right way!

Never cook vegetables with butter, excessive oil, cream or in the deep fryer. Instead, try a splash of lemon juice, a drizzle of balsamic vinegar, or a twist of black pepper before oven-baking vegetables like cauliflower or sweet potatoes. Leave out the pads of butter from recipes like curried carrots — the rich spices already give the carrots a great flavor without the added calories and saturated fat. Experiment and you'll find that many vegetables, like tomatoes and bell peppers, are delicious when baked or blackened on a grill, without adding much of anything. Remember, the fewer ingredients the better when it comes to keeping vegetables low-fat and low-calorie.

### Have whole fruits instead of juices

Whole fruits can help you lose weight because they contain essential phytonutrients, and their fiber and water content help you feel satisfied. On the flip side, commercial fruit juice usually includes added sugars and 100 or more calories per glass. Also, when the pulp and skin of the fruit is removed, the sugar absorbs quickly within the body and can cause cravings later in the day. Juicing removes the bulk of the fruit so juice does not fill you up like the real fruit does. Half of a large grapefruit has 50 calories, 2 grams of fiber, and 11 grams of sugar, while 8 fluid ounces of grapefruit juice contains about 100 calories and 22 grams of sugar. When you're craving something sweet and juicy, reach for the real piece of fruit rather than sugary juice. For a dessert substitute, try putting pineapple slices or halved peaches on the grill for a warm, sweet treat without high fructose corn syrup and added calories.

To save hundreds of calories and dozens of grams of fat, ask for oil and vinegar. A few splashes of balsamic or red wine vinegar are often all you need on a vegetable salad. Even better? Squeeze a fresh lemon over your salad for a zero-calorie dressing.

### Pass on ready-made grocery store salads

When you're cutting calories, pass on ready-made grocery store salads from the deli aisle. Typical choices — English pea, pasta, potato, Waldorf, macaroni, broccoli, chicken, tuna, and egg salads — are all full of mayo. It's what holds these salads together, giving them their consistency. These are not healthy sides. They are not "salads" like you want them to be

— "salads" meaning fresh, healthy, and satisfying. A better choice that you can make on your own in a hurry: fruit salad. Chop a banana, apple, and red grapes, and add a can of drained mandarin oranges. Sprinkle cinnamon over the top and you have enough to feed 2 to 4 people a sweet side salad with no fat and only natural sugars. Another healthier, lighter option is to make tuna salad Mediterranean style, with chopped celery, olives, olive oil, lemon juice, and salt and pepper.

> A favorite diet secret is substituting Greek or other non-fat yogurt for sour cream and mayo. You won't lose any of the creaminess but with zero grams of fat and packed with protein, you're making a smart trade-off.

## Enjoy a delicious bowl of soup

Warm liquids not only help calm and relax the body, they provide a sense of satiation because they must be ingested slowly. Thus, vegetable soup is a great weight-loss food. Soup is relatively low in calories per serving, and the high water content sends messages to your brain that you're full. You'll have to slow down while eating the hot soup, and bites are always a spoonful. Have a tomato-based soup with high-fiber whole grains, beans, vegetables, and/or lean meat. If the bowl is small, pair it with a turkey sandwich on whole wheat bread (hold the mayo to eliminate extra calories). The numerous ingredients will take time to digest and leave you feeling full longer. Avoid cream-based soups since they contain butter and fat, and are high in calories.

## Incorporate veggies in unexpected ways

Not everyone who wants to lose weight also enjoys eating vegetables. Even people who love veggies typically don't eat enough of them! Rather than sitting down with a pile of produce and forcing yourself to eat it, try sneaking vegetables into dishes you already love. You won't even notice they're there, and you'll be getting the nutrients and fiber you need to lose weight and stay healthy. Some great ideas for incorporating vegetables in unexpected ways include pureeing carrots and zucchini in marinara sauce, meatballs, and burger patties; adding sweet potatoes to pancake batter; substituting baked butternut squash for pasta in mac 'n' cheese; and using steamed cauliflower in mashed potatoes. Vegetables are a crucial part of losing weight, because they are fiber-dense but low in calories, so they fill you up longer for fewer calories. Plus, veggies are packed with natural minerals and vitamins to ward off illness and disease. Just because you're a former steak-and-potatoes type or you're trying to cook for a family that refuses to eat their vegetables doesn't mean you can't get the nutrients and fiber your body craves to lose weight.

Warm liquids not only help calm and relax the body, they provide a sense of satiation because they must be ingested slowly. Thus, vegetable soup is a great weight-loss food.

## Satisfy a sweet tooth with spices

There are many ways you can satisfy a sweet tooth without cookies, cakes, candy, or ice cream. The urge for something sweet can often be satisfied when you add spices to certain foods. Add the spices commonly found in desserts — vanilla, cinnamon, nutmeg, clove, ginger, and allspice — to other foods that are already naturally sweet, such as baked apples, pears, peaches, and sweet potatoes. You can achieve the flavors and sweetness you crave from baked goods without all the extra sugar, fat, and calories.

## Find a low-calorie alternative to your daily latte

Unless you specify, coffee drinks are made with 2% milk, which adds fat, calories, and carbs to your beverage. Additionally, any sweetener, such as flavored syrups, caramel, or cocoa powder, add dozens of calories and carbs as well. And specialty drinks typically include whipped cream, chocolate shavings and other high-calorie toppings. Even if you opt for a light or "skinny" version of your favorite latte, you're looking at 200 calories.

**Trim Up to 300 Calories!**
**Pass:** Granola with raisins
**Swap:** Turkey pepperoni instead of salami pepperoni

If you can't live without coffee, the key to losing weight is to go as pared down as possible with your selections. Start with hot or iced Café Americano (a.k.a, regular coffee). Sounds dull? It doesn't have to be! One or two pumps of sugar-free flavored syrup can jazz it up. A splash of nonfat milk is reasonable. Cinnamon is also a favorite coffee condiment of many dieters. It packs lots of flavor without the added sugar. Making this switch will let you start your day with under 25 calories per medium coffee, creating a 100-calorie-plus deficit right from the start of your day.

## Don't dip into fat and calories

Dips are popular at barbecues, potlucks, and housewarming parties, but most — spinach and artichoke, French onion, 7-layer bean dip — are jam-packed with fat and calories in every spoonful. Most of the most popular party dips are the creamy and cheesy versions, which have 200 calories or more per ¼-cup serving, more than 10 grams of fat, and include several grams of saturated fat.

If you're attending or hosting a party, skip the veggie tray from the grocery store, which almost always includes Ranch dressing. Buy veggies individually (usually cheaper than the pre-made tray anyhow), such as grape tomatoes, celery sticks, bell peppers, cauliflower and snap peas, and make your own healthy dip. A great one, even for the cooking-challenged, is hummus, which is just chickpeas, olive oil, tahini, lemon juice, garlic, as well as black and cayenne pepper blended to a smooth texture in a food processor. Or to make Mediterranean layered dip, a perfect substitute for high-calorie bean dip, you can stack low-fat Greek yogurt, kalamata olives, feta, tomatoes, red pepper, cucumbers, garlic, and whatever else you like. Top it with chopped romaine lettuce and sprinkle paprika over the top for a healthy, hearty alternative.

## Eat more natural peanut butter!

Natural peanut butter is a truly amazing diet food! It has heart-healthy monounsaturated fats and doesn't include the hydrogenated oils, sweeteners, and extra salt of other peanut butters. You'll notice the label on natural peanut butter includes only two ingredients: peanuts and salt. It's a great food for losing weight because it maintains blood sugar levels and has fiber to keep you feeling full longer. Instead of a high-calorie muffin for breakfast, eat two tablespoons of peanut butter on whole wheat toast. And peanut butter on a banana or apple makes a great snack. Although it might have as many calories as a bag of chips, not all calories are created equal. Peanut butter's fiber and healthy fats keep you full longer so you'll eat less throughout the day.

> All-natural peanut butter is a great food for losing weight because it maintains blood sugar levels and has fiber to keep you feeling full longer. Instead of a high-calorie muffin for breakfast, eat two tablespoons of peanut butter on whole wheat toast.

## Don't mess up the most important meal of the day

Yes, you need to eat breakfast — but it's what you eat that is going to help you or keep you from losing weight. *Parade* magazine's annual report, "What America Really Eats," found that breakfast is actually becoming the highest calorie meal of the day for many people. That's because breakfast sandwiches and burritos — generally made with bacon, ham, cheese, fried potatoes, and eggs made the top 10 on both men and women's lists of most-ordered menu items last year. Unfortunately, these items typically contain between 400 and 800 calories (not including the latte or orange juice you're probably washing them down with).

A better choice for weight loss? Protein-packed eggs. A study from the Pennington Biomedical Research Center showed that participants who ate 2 eggs for breakfast lost 65 percent more weight than participants who ate a bagel, even though the bagel and the eggs contained an equal number of calories. The egg-eaters also reported feeling more energetic than the participants who ate the bagels. Now, you do need some carbs, but make sure they're complex carbs such a whole wheat English muffin or oatmeal (without all the sugary toppings). Complex carbs make you feel full and burn directly into energy.

> A great weight-loss food? Protein-packed eggs. A study from the Pennington Biomedical Research Center showed that participants who ate 2 eggs for breakfast lost 65 percent more weight than participants who ate a bagel, even though the bagel and the eggs contained an equal number of calories.

## Beware of low-fat products

A report called "Can Low-Fat Nutrition Labels Lead to Obesity," published in the *Journal of Marketing Research*, offered a dose of reality as to why so many people don't lose a single pound from eating low-fat or fat-free foods. The study found that both normal-weight and overweight participants ate more when presented with a low-fat option of a nutrient-poor and calorie-rich snack food. Additionally, they found that overweight participants were more inclined than normal-weight people to overindulge. Why? The study contends that low-fat food labels increase consumption because they decrease guilt and give the false perception that you can eat more of the item. And it seemed that this was particularly true for overweight subjects.

In a portion of this study conducted at a university open house, 2 gallon-size bowls of M&M's were set out, one labeled "New Colors of Regular M&M's" and the other labeled "New 'Low-Fat' M&M's" (although no such low-fat product currently exists). As expected, participants ate more M&M's (28.4 percent more!) when they were labeled as low-fat than when they were labeled as regular. Furthermore, overweight participants took 16 percent more M&M's than normal-weight participants. While all participants increased their consumption, overweight subjects ate an average of 90 additional calories more of the candies labeled as "low-fat."

Don't love veggies? Try sneaking them into dishes you already love. You won't even notice they're there, and you'll be getting the nutrients and fiber you need to lose weight and stay healthy.

# 09

"Never go backward. Attempt,
and do it with all your might."

~ Charles Simmons

# Eat Smart While Dining Out

A recent survey found that the majority of dieters said that dining out represented the biggest challenge to their weight loss. While able to stick to their eating plan at home, at work, and even at friends' houses, once in a restaurant, their goals and willpower quickly unraveled. Why does dining out present such a challenge to so many people? One reason is that restaurant food is cooked primarily with your palate in mind, not your waistline. Indeed, chefs go to great lengths to include sauces, batters, and other calorie-laden accessories to dishes to improve their flavor and presentation.

Because you cannot control the meal's ingredients, you may end up eating far more calories than you would like. Statistics show that people eat an average of 500 calories more when dining out than at home. For example, if you made yourself a hamburger at home, you might choose a low-fat burger, or maybe even substitute it with a turkey or veggie burger. You might choose a low-fat or multi-grain bun, skip the cheese, and serve it with a small side salad. But in a restaurant, you will be served a giant burger, up to a half-pound in size. The burger could be topped with special sauces, cheese, and bacon and served with potato salad or fries on the side. Once these items are in front of you, you'll surely be tempted to eat them.

To compound the problem, restaurant portions in the U.S. have nearly tripled in size over the last few decades. Have you ever heard someone who traveled abroad complain about the small portion sizes in Europe? That's because in Italy, for example, meat, pasta, and vegetables are ordered and served as individual courses, whereas Americans are used to having all three come piled high in the same dish. In the U.S., you're eating far more at a restaurant than you would if you were cooking for yourself at home. A recent study showed that people consume 50 percent more calories, fat, and sodium when they eat out. Therefore, when dining out you must make an extra effort to control the ingredients and portion size of the meal you order the same way you would when cooking at home. Don't be embarrassed to inquire about how something is prepared or served, and ask for substitutions if necessary. And you never need to feel like you have to eat everything on your plate. The "clean plate" rule of your childhood no longer needs to apply!

Finally, as this chapter discusses, restaurant menus have been set up to make food sound as appealing as possible, and many have photos as well. The name of the "Molten Chocolate Lava Cake with Crème Fraîche" already sounds delicious, but when coupled with a photo, it's all you can do not to order one to enjoy all by yourself. And if the menu doesn't tempt you enough, the servers at restaurants have been coached to sell you certain dishes, drinks, and desserts.

Luckily, American restaurants are finally beginning to accommodate the public's newfound interest in losing weight. National chains and fast food restaurants now offer healthy or low-calorie dishes that help the calorie-conscious have a pleasant dining experience. And as part of the 2010 national health care reform bill, any fast food or chain restaurant with 20 or more locations will be required to post calorie counts right on menus, menu boards, and even drive-thrus. The idea is that with the nutritional information right in front of you, clueless eaters and calorie-counters alike will be able to make smart choices that eliminate hundreds of calories.

*You never need to feel like you have to eat everything on your plate. The "clean plate" rule of your childhood no longer needs to apply!*

## Don't starve yourself all day before dining out

Don't make the common mistake of barely eating all day in anticipation of dinner with friends. You'll be starving come dinner time and you'll overeat. Instead, eat normally throughout the day and have a small snack before you leave for your dinner. According to Purdue University research, eating a handful of peanuts about an hour before dinner will cause you to eat less total calories and fat during your main meal. Or, in case you don't have a chance to eat prior to your meal, order a broth-based soup or small side salad as a starter. Both contain about 150 calories, will fill you up, and lead you to eat less of your main meal.

## Decide what to order ahead of time

Before you leave for a restaurant, check the online menu and decide on a few options that you can order and still work toward your target calorie deficit. Many locations now offer their nutritional facts online, but if your eatery doesn't, some safe bets are chicken, fish, or lean steak with vegetables. Look out for creamy sauces and sugary marinades and glazes. If you decide ahead of time what you're going to order, you won't be easily swayed into sharing an appetizer or high-calorie entrée once you're surrounded by friends.

### Say bye-bye to the bread basket

A fast place to eliminate 100 calories or more is to stay away from the bread basket when dining out. Although you might be able to resist the rolls through willpower alone, asking the waiter to remove the bread basket from the table is more foolproof. If you were trying to quit drinking, you'd stay away from bars, right? The same goes for losing weight. Carbohydrate addiction is a real problem for many struggling dieters, because eating carbs spikes insulin and lowers blood sugar, creating the desire for even more carbs. Don't put temptation in front of you! Have the bread basket removed or, if the people you are dining with want to keep the bread basket, ask that it be moved to the far end of the table out of your immediate reach.

## Beware of "healthy" restaurant menus

Meeting friends or coworkers at Chili's, Olive Garden, or Cheesecake Factory seems like a good idea — large menus with something for everyone — but they're precarious spots for someone trying to cut calories. In an attempt to appeal to people watching their calories, many restaurants have started offering "healthy" menus — Applebee's has a 550-calorie-or-less menu, Cheesecake Factory's Weight Management selections all have 600 calories or less, and Macaroni Grill recently underwent a complete menu revamp that offers healthier choices. However, a 600-calorie lunch isn't the best fit for a low-calorie plan like *Lose Weight Fast Diet*. You want to aim for around 400 calories per main meal. Plus, these menus only really account for calories, so many of the items are super-high in fat, sugar, and carbs. For example, the "Weight Management Asian Chicken Salad" from Cheesecake Factory contains 574 calories, 39 grams of fat, 68 grams of carbs, and 20 grams of sugar! You're better off sticking to meals with the fewest number of ingredients possible: grilled salmon (watch for any glazes and ask for it without them), brown rice, and steamed veggies, for instance.

Before you leave for a restaurant, check the online menu and decide on a few options that you can order and still work toward your target calorie deficit. Don't wait until you arrive, when your eyes may be bigger than your stomach.

### Don't worry about what others think of what you order

When dining out, many people are so worried about what others are thinking that they order only a small side salad, only to overeat or binge on junk food later when they're alone. When they finally get to eat in the privacy of their own homes, they feel relieved and comforted by the food.

Anxiety while dining out is most prevalent in women, who often worry about being judged for eating or not appearing "ladylike" to others. "When I eat in a group, I am convinced that everyone is thinking, 'Why is she eating so much? She doesn't need to eat that,'" said one woman who admits to this behavior. But you cannot let food control you! While it is important to exert self-control when you are eating in a group, don't let others' opinions or what they are eating affect you. Stick to your diet plan, don't give in to food peer pressure, and enjoy your meal. Your company won't be assessing what or how much you ate or didn't eat — they will appreciate that you have a healthy relationship with food.

## Don't give in to eating peer pressure

You may feel like the relaxed, social atmosphere of going out to eat with friends makes it difficult to refuse a dessert or drink. You're afraid your friends will think you're not fun if you turn down food or alcohol. It's very true that social settings create peer pressure, even among friends. People who feel the need to eat to please others or fit in will always eat more in social situations. Instead, save hundreds of calories by saying a firm "No thanks" when your dinner companions suggest splitting an appetizer or dessert. Alcohol and coffee drinks also rack up major calories, so order hot tea if everyone is having after-dinner drinks. If someone questions you, just say you don't feel like drinking alcohol and leave it at that. Remind yourself that no one will remember who ate what an hour after the meal, so stick to your calorie budget for that meal and never feel pressured to overindulge.

## Get out of the buffet line

Buffets are tempting because of the value, the wide selection of food, and the option to go for seconds. It can be extremely difficult to practice self-control while eating a single dish, let alone resist the wide array of food, drinks, and desserts presented at buffets! The standard buffet has over 100 different options. The uncontrolled variety at buffets and the mentality that you can eat as much as you want can derail the most disciplined eater.

Avoid buffet restaurants, and if the place you're dining out offers a buffet special to accompany their menu, always opt to order from the menu.

## Veggies on the side can't be buttered or fried

Just because you chose the side of vegetables over the side of French fries, don't pat yourself on the back quite yet. A side of vegetables is only the low-calorie option if you insist on having them prepared the right way. Unfortunately, the easiest way for restaurants to cook typical side-dish veggies like zucchini, carrots, and broccoli is to sauté them in butter and salt. It's a bad sign when vegetables come served on a small side plate — they're probably soaking in butter. The extra plate keeps the melted butter runoff contained and separate from your main meal. Veggies bathed in butter or battered and fried mean hundreds of extra calories and tons of saturated fat.

People who feel the need to eat to please others or fit in will always eat more in social situations. Instead, save hundreds of calories by saying a firm "No thanks" when your dinner companions suggest splitting an appetizer or dessert.

To keep them healthy and delicious, ask for your veggies steamed, sautéed in a touch of olive oil, or roasted. Don't feel guilty about sending them back if they come prepared in an unhealthy way! And when you cook them at home, try a splash of lemon juice, a drizzle of balsamic vinegar, or a twist of black pepper before oven-baking vegetables like cauliflower or sweet potatoes.

## Resist the sales pitch

Servers are trained to describe their dishes in very appealing terms. Plus, many restaurants offer employees bonuses if they sell non-entrée items such as dessert, appetizers, and specialty drinks. For example, instead of asking, "What would you like to drink?" they may say, "We have a frozen strawberry margarita that would be perfect with some chips and guacamole." Or a server may bring by a dessert tray or drop off a dessert menu with tempting photos without even being asked. Restaurants know hunger is very visual, so seeing a slice of cake often translates into ordering it. Don't fall into this trap that ends up adding hundreds of extra calories to your day. Politely tell your sever that you are not interested in looking at the dessert menu and not to bring the dessert tray by. Stick to your game plan and order only the items that stay within your calorie budget.

Enjoy the company of friends while eating healthy by hosting a dinner party where you cook a majority of the dishes and provide the beverages. Organizing a group meal in your home means consuming hundreds of calories less than if you were heading out to a restaurant.

## Host your own dinner party

Enjoy the company of friends while eating healthy by hosting a dinner party where you cook a majority of the dishes and provide the beverages. Cooking at home means eating smaller portions and up to 50 percent fewer calories than you would at a restaurant, and you can control what goes into each dish. This is a big benefit when you consider that many restaurant meals are prepared with unhealthy oils, butter, and creamy sauces. Serve courses that include fruits, vegetables, lean meats, and whole grains, such as recipes taken from Mediterranean cuisine. Serve natural sparkling water, like Perrier, with several choices of garnish to avoid the empty calories of alcohol. Guests can feel free to bring wine or beer, but you'll have an option for sticking to your weight-loss program. Organizing a group meal in your home means consuming hundreds of calories less than if you were heading out to a restaurant, and you can still spend an evening socializing with friends.

# 10

"Success means having the courage, the determination, and the will to become the person you believe you were meant to be."

~ George A. Sheehan

# The Secrets of Slim People

**Do you have a friend who always passes on dessert,** while you count down the minutes to treating yourself to a cookie or ice cream at the end of the day? What about someone in your family who loses 10 pounds without even trying, while you struggle with all your might just to lose a couple of pounds? It seems that all of us know at least one person who has an easy time losing weight, or even more infuriating, someone who is so naturally thin that he or she has never even had to think about it at all! Part of this person's easy relationship with their weight can be attributed to genes; indeed, some of us simply inherit high metabolic rates or extremely lean and muscular body types, which offer natural weight-loss advantages.

Yet naturally slender people also tend to have different lifestyles than those who need to actively try to lose weight. They are less likely to use food as an emotional crutch or to resort to eating when bored, nervous, or tired. They are also more likely to be naturally drawn to physical activities that keep their metabolisms high and their muscles working. Most important,

## Stay Motivated!

"Make the most of yourself, for that is
all there is of you."
~ Ralph Waldo Emerson

they tend to think differently about hunger, and thus make different choices when considering what foods to eat, when to eat them, and how much of them to eat.

What works for naturally thin people can also work for you as you continue to change your habits and lifestyle. Genetics do play a role; however, adopting the habits of thin, healthy individuals can help you to lose 10 pounds easier and faster than you thought possible. Take the negative connotations away from the word "diet" and think of this program, instead, as mimicking the powerful and proven habits of slim, healthy people.

Never fall into the fad-diet trap, however. Celebrity or Hollywood diets, system cleanses, and outlandish weight-loss claims sound too good to be true — because they are. Fad diets aren't a lifestyle, they're a quick fix, and even then, many won't give you any results. And the ones that do aren't healthy. It isn't smart or wise to eat nothing but grapefruit or cereal for 2 meals of the day. You won't be getting the energy and nutrients you need, you'll feel sluggish, and you'll put the weight right back on when you're done with the fad diet. When you read health magazines, pay little attention to ads for fad diets or articles on celebrity weight loss and look for the "real reader success stories." These men and women have generally lost weight in a healthy way and have continued to keep it off. These are the diets and workout tips to model yourself after. These formerly overweight individuals have learned just what you will in this chapter: how to eat, exercise, and think like a thin person.

## Choose being satisfied over being stuffed

Most people who are able to maintain their weight finish eating when they feel neither hungry nor full. Those who are overweight tend to continue eating past the point of comfort. The next time you eat, periodically stop and put down your utensils. Notice how your stomach feels. Can you stop eating now and feel satisfied? Find out if it is true hunger or habit that is driving you to finish your meal. If you are used to eating past the point of comfort, gradually cut back on portions, and eat more slowly until you get used to stopping at a comfortable level.

## Don't view hunger as good or bad

Hunger is just your body's natural signal to fuel itself. People tend to read into their hunger more than they need to. Thin people look at hunger as a simple signal from their bodies that they need food for energy. People who overeat and are overweight tend to either look forward to every meal, snack, and treat or completely dread every time they eat, fretting over every calorie. They consistently overeat or eat even when they don't have any physical signals to do so. Thin people recognize their hunger and understand where these sensations are coming from. If you find yourself eating for no reason, try skipping a snack. You may realize that you didn't even need it.

> People who overeat tend to either look forward to every meal, snack, and treat or completely dread every time they eat, fretting over every calorie. They eat even when they don't have any physical signals to do so. Thin people look at food as fuel and recognize their hunger and understand where these sensations are coming from.

## Eat more fruit

A study based on the nutritional habits of slim people showed that they have an additional serving of fruit, consume more fiber, and have less fat per day than people who are overweight. The additional serving of fruit may account for the difference in weight since fruit is naturally low in fat and high in fiber. Its bulk and sweetness may satisfy lean people with a lot less calories than the cookies and pastries consumed by heavier individuals. Try to include at least 3 to 5 servings of fruit each day. Keep easy-to-eat fruits that are low on the glycemic index — meaning they cause the smallest changes to blood sugar and insulin levels — in visible places in your kitchen and office so they are handy for when you need a snack. Grapefruit, apples, cherries, and pears are great choices.

## Exercise an important muscle — your self control

One of the most significant behavioral indicators of weight is the amount of self-control a person has. Studies show that people who have fine-tuned their self-restraint have the lowest BMI. On the flip side, a low level of restraint has been linked to weight gain of up to 30 pounds. Your willpower is just like a muscle in that it gets stronger the more you use it! Learn to control your appetite. Plan ahead for situations where you have traditionally lacked self-control, such as celebrations and social events. Decide in advance what you will and will not eat. Pass on alcohol since it lowers inhibitions. You can't always control what is served; your willpower is sometimes all you've got.

## Don't tempt yourself!

You're tying to burn or cut a significant number of calories a day to lose up to 10 pounds, so now is not the time to be testing your willpower. Don't tempt yourself by strolling through the frozen pizza section or chip and soda aisles at the grocery store. You know what your triggers are by now, be it baked goods or the grab-and-go candy bars at the supermarket checkout. Don't spend *any* time in those aisles. If you must be in the area, don't linger, and put your "bad-food blinders" on. Get what you need and move on. And don't push the limits by thinking you'll have just a few bites of birthday cake or just 1 or 2 cookies from a package. Eating the fatty, sugary foods you love sends pleasure signals to your brain and stopping at just a bite or two will be nearly impossible. Why take the risk?

## Get moving!

Studies indicate that slim people move around several hours a week more than those who are overweight. This extra activity can account for an additional weight loss of 2 to 3 pounds! How much do you move around during the day? If you have a desk job, you might spend a large portion of your day sitting — although you don't have to. Get up and move around as

Keep easy-to-eat fruits that are low on the glycemic index — meaning they cause the smallest changes to blood sugar and insulin levels — in visible places in your kitchen and office so they are handy for when you need a snack. Grapefruit, apples, cherries, and pears are great choices.

much as you can. Walk around while talking on the phone; take the stairs up and down a few times; walk to the other side of the office to talk to a coworker in person, rather than sending an email. Your day should involve taking 10,000 steps a day. This type of activity is extremely valuable to your body's "non-exercise activity thermogenesis," or NEAT, which is the calorie burning process that happens naturally from everyday movements, including standing up, fidgeting, turning, bending, and walking. A physically active person burns approximately 30 percent of their calories through daily "non-intentional exercise," versus 15 percent for sedentary people. Try to incorporate other physical activities into your day, such as vacuuming, shopping, or playing with your kids or dog.

### Ask yourself, is it worth it?

Thin people evaluate what they eat based on how hard they will have to exercise to burn off the extra calories. If you are considering splurging on a piece of cheesecake, for instance, consider that you'll need to run for 45 minutes to get back to where your calorie count was prior to eating it. That's just to break even! And when you're looking to create a calorie deficit each day, you'll be way behind if you have that dessert. Ask yourself, do you want to negate a good, sweaty gym session with a few bites of food? Think thin and say no to any snack, drink, or treat that will mean extra hours of exercise (or depriving yourself of nutritious food) to compensate. In the end, you'll realize it just isn't worth it.

### Get some ZZZZZs

Statistically, people who have less body fat get about 2 more hours of sleep a week versus those who are overweight. Researchers suggest that increased body weight from lack of sleep is linked to our hormones. Sleep deprivation decreases the amounts of leptin in our system, the hormone that suppresses hunger, and increases the levels of ghrelin, an appetite-boosting hormone. Cravings for salty and sugary foods increase and motivation to stay away from high-calorie foods decreases. Thin people tend to get between 7 and 9 hours of sleep a night. Give yourself the best shot at a great day of healthy eating by going to bed 15 to 30 minutes earlier than your typical bedtime. If you have trouble settling into bed, a warm bath or mug of non-caffeinated tea can help (warm liquids are soothing). Also, be sure to put away your electronics 30 minutes before you get into bed. Checking emails, browsing the Internet, and text messaging can make it hard to fall asleep.

## Don't forget about your diet on the weekends

A physically active person burns approximately 30 percent of their calories through daily "non-intentional exercise," versus 15 percent for sedentary people.

People who maintain their weight follow their diet game plan 7 days a week. Saturdays and Sundays aren't free rein to forget about smart eating and overindulge. To lose significant weight each week, you need to resist lazy-weekend temptations: beer-soaked sporting events, late night pizza binges, and calorie-packed pancake brunches. Too often you'll hear dieters call one day of the week their "cheat day," but consider that eating an extra 500 calories on Saturday may mean having to create a 2,000-calorie deficit on another day. It's just not smart or healthy. Maintaining similar eating patterns for all days of the week will help you establish healthy choices as long-term habits. Don't forget to plan your meals for the entire week ahead of time. This will keep you from wavering from your eating plan on the weekends.

## Always ask for dressing on the side

As a rule of thumb: Don't ever trust restaurant salad dressings! Smart eaters know that even the light-sounding dressings on restaurant menus, such as raspberry vinaigrette or Asian sesame vinaigrette, are full of sugar. And restaurants are infamous for pouring on far too much dressing. A weight-loss tip: Dip your fork into the dressing cup several times and spread it over the salad. You'll get the flavor of the dressing without soaking your salad and adding tons of calories. And, if you don't douse your salad with a full cup of dressing, you can take part of it home to eat that night or the next day.

Thin people learn to tune out food advertisements and stick with their eating plans no matter what special combo meal is now available. Be aware of how food ads affect you, and you'll be one step closer to thinking thin and putting an end to mindless snacking.

## Tune out advertising

Online, on TV, or simply driving down the road, you are exposed to dozens of advertisements for food each day. An interesting study from the Yale Rudd Center for Food Policy and Obesity showed that people are profoundly affected by food advertising, and that these effects occur regardless of people's initial hunger. The study measured the amount of snack foods consumed during and after advertising exposure and found that both children and adults consumed significantly more of both healthy and unhealthy snack foods following exposure to advertising. Additionally, food advertising increased consumption of all available foods, even foods that were not presented in the advertisements, contradicting food industry claims that advertising affects only brand preferences and not overall nutrition. Jennifer Harris, one of the authors of the study, concluded, "Food advertising triggers automatic eating, regardless of hunger, and is a significant contributor to the obesity epidemic."

Stay alert when food advertisements pop up around you. Thin people learn to tune them out and stick with their eating plans, no matter what special combo meal is now available at a neighborhood restaurant. Observe correlations between snacking, emotional hunger, and advertisements. Be aware of how food ads affect you, and you'll be one step closer to thinking thin and putting an end to mindless snacking.

Statistically, people who have less body fat get about 2 more hours of sleep a week versus those who are overweight.

### Practice positive visualization

Ask yourself, "What is stopping me from losing weight?" Do you believe you're doomed to fail? Do you start your diet imagining all the foods you'll miss or how hungry you'll be? Healthy, fit people look at eating well and exercising as a lifestyle, not a punishment or a constant battle. Practice being positive about your new program from the get-go. Disassociate your eating plan with restriction and deprivation. Instead, view it as enjoying the right foods in the right amounts. Now, visualize your happier, healthier, thinner self after losing weight. Picture yourself in a swimsuit, lying in the warm sun on the beach, feeling confident. Visualize yourself cooking and enjoying a healthy dinner with friends or family. Imagine yourself walking into a party full of people and how they'll all notice your new body, confidence, and happiness. You can already feel how proud you will be. Positive visualization reinforces the reasons you're losing weight and keeps your eye on the prize.

# 11

"Self-image sets the boundaries of individual accomplishment."

~ Maxwell Maltz

# Exercising to Lose Weight

**Too many people falsely believe** they can lose weight by simply eating less or eating better, without sweating one bit. However, creating a calorie deficit from your diet alone, without integrating exercise, is nearly impossible, if not dangerous. In addition, an extremely low-calorie diet means you'll lack the energy and stamina you need to get through your day. On the flip side, many people assume if they become moderately active they can lose weight without giving up their indulgences of ice cream, burritos, and burgers. Unfortunately, neither is a healthy approach, and neither will allow you to lose 10 pounds or reach your ideal weight.

Consider this: A University of Virginia study reported that to lose 1 pound of body fat you would have to do 250,000 sit-ups — or 100 sit-ups every day for 7 years. Exercise alone won't give you a flat stomach and defined abs — it's the layer of body fat covering your muscles that needs to be whittled away through eating low-fat, low-calorie foods, and cardiovascular work that allows muscles to show.

Likewise, a Mayo Clinic report revealed the prevalence of "skinny overweight" people, or what is being called "normal weight obesity." As many as 30 million "thin" Americans are believed to have a body fat percentage that puts them in the overweight category and at risk for disease, despite appearing to be of a normal weight.

Healthy eating and exercise are a powerful fat and disease-fighting combo, and only with the combination of the two can you drop unwanted pounds and start feeling amazing.

The *Lose Weight Fast Diet* covers the importance of redefining your food choices, creating a game plan to address each meal and craving, and making healthy changes to your habits. This knowledge will help you eat hundreds of calories less a day and shed unwanted pounds; however, you can't lose weight, and keep it off, without exercise. You need to stay full and satisfied throughout the day. Cutting calories through diet restriction alone may very well mean you're eating too little, and eating too little leaves the door dangerously open for bingeing. However, including exercise in your weight-loss program means you can easily reach a substantial calorie deficit without starving yourself. Just an hour of exercise a day burns hundreds of calories, making meeting your goal very doable. In addition, you will find that exercise is energizing, builds muscle tone, curbs your appetite, and increases your metabolism.

So what is the best exercise regimen for you to embark on? The answer depends on your personality, interests, and individual abilities. You can do it all at once or integrate it into 2 or 3 segments over the course of your day. Just be sure to build a plan that fits into your daily calendar, and keep in mind that the common ingredient for any successful exercise program is to choose activities you will enjoy doing and that you may even look forward to every day.

## Incorporate all 3 elements of fitness

Your fitness program should include all 3 essential elements for successful weight loss and maintenance: cardiovascular activities to burn calories, benefit your heart and reduce body fat; resistance or strength training for muscle tone; and a basic stretching routine to improve flexibility and prevent injury. Cardio is the most beneficial for weight loss and should be your main focus, but each element complements the others. Resistance and strength training will firm up muscles as the unwanted pounds melt away. Increased muscle mass will also burn extra calories throughout the day. Stretching and flexibility develop range of motion, increase muscle elasticity, achieve muscle balance, and protect the body from injury.

When you do cardio, you want to make sure you're moving continuously and getting your heart rate up. You should be breathing hard. The rule of thumb is, be working hard enough during cardio that you can answer questions but not carry on a conversation. Typical activities include jogging/running, elliptical training, bicycling/spinning, and cardio classes such as step aerobics, kickboxing, and aerobic dance. For strength training, aim for at least two 30-minute sessions per week that may include free weights, weight machines, resistance equipment, muscular endurance training, and toning activities such as power yoga or Pilates. Focus on activities that exercise each of the major muscle groups or work more than one muscle group at the same time. Stretching is important before, during, and after a workout. A study found that regular stretching can increase your strength by up to 19 percent when interspersed between weight-training exercises, for instance. Try doing 10 or 15 minutes of basic Ashtanga yoga poses.

## Did You Know?

One of the best predictors of maintaining a fitness program over time is exercising in a social environment, like a gym or fitness class, or having a workout buddy. Think about it: The people you see each time you exercise become friends and acquaintances who expect to say hello to you, so you're less likely to skip a class or workout. Plus, you're making new friends while you slim down!

## Create a realistic schedule you can stick to

Schedule your workouts at the beginning of the week, just like you are doing with your meals for the week. Be realistic! If you're not a morning person, don't schedule 6 a.m. runs. If you like to relax after work, don't pretend you're going to take a yoga class in the evenings. Take a look at your calendar and pencil in workouts for at least 5 days of the week, on days and times that are most doable. For instance, plan morning workouts for the days when you'll want to meet friends after work, or schedule a lunchtime hike for a day when you want to sleep in. Building exercise around your personal schedule and lifestyle means you're more likely to meet your goals.

## Get a walking workout

Many people starting out a fitness plan turn to good old-fashioned walking. On a nice day, consider a stroll around your neighborhood. In cold or rainy weather, go to the mall and log miles while you window shop. Walking is a cost-effective activity that simply requires a good pair of shoes. Walking may sound too good to be true, but it is an aerobic activity that burns calories. Consider the fact that for a 150-pound person, walking at 2 mph, which is approximately a 30-minute mile, burns 189 calories per hour. Walking a 20-minute mile at a 3 mph pace uses 300 calories per hour. Walking a moderate, 15-minute mile for an average of 4 mph burns 300 calories per hour. The faster you walk, the more calories you will burn.

Look at your weekly schedule and be realistic! If you're not a morning person, don't schedule 6 a.m. runs. If you like to relax after work, don't pretend you're going to take a yoga class in the evenings.

If you're not sure how far a mile is in your neighborhood, you can drive your car while looking at your odometer or buy a small pedometer to count your steps. The U.S. Surgeon General has recommended walking 30 minutes daily to strive toward a weekly goal of 10,000 steps, or roughly 5 miles. Those on a weight-loss program should strive for a minimum of 12,000 to 15,000 steps, which should take about 45 minutes per day.

## Fend off food cravings with exercise

To increase your daily exercise as well as stave off cravings and hunger pangs, go for a walk the next time you feel like eating when it's not a snack or meal time. People often snack when they need a break from work or family, or when they're bored. Instead, try going for a 15-minute walk and allow the craving to pass. Walking for 15 minutes will burn 75 calories for a 150-pound person. So instead of eating a 150-calorie snack out of boredom, you'll have actually burned calories!

## Find solutions to your exorcise excuses

There are many excuses to skip exercise or to let a fitness plan fall by the wayside after a short time. But you won't be able to lose weight without exercise to complement a reduced-calorie diet. Get out a piece of paper and write down the reasons you've been avoiding exercise, joining a gym, or taking a fitness class. Some of the most common reasons people use to avoid physical activity include:

"I don't have the time."
"I'm too tired and I don't feel like it."
"I'm not very good at exercising."
"It's not convenient to get to my workout place."
"I'm afraid and embarrassed."
"It's too expensive to join a gym."

Now write down solutions to these excuses. For example, if your number one reason for skipping exercise is "I don't have time," use half your lunch break to go for a brisk walk or take a bike ride with your family instead of seeing a movie (you'll still spend time together, get to interact, and do something good for everyone's health). The bottom line is, there is never a good excuse to be sedentary. There are great gyms and fitness facilities of all types and price ranges. If you find the traditional gym environment isn't for you, try a cycling club or dance class. If money is a concern, sign up for a hiking club — things like hiking, swimming, and rollerblading are always free. There are hundreds of ways to burn calories, so stop making excuses — make time and find something you like to do.

## Take measures to avoid injury

Nothing puts a cramp in your weight loss like an injury. And if it's something serious enough, it can even mean the end of your exercise plan all together. There are several ways to avoid injury when you're embarking on a new fitness plan. Always warm up and cool down for at least 5 to 10 minutes, before and after workouts. Warm up is especially important if you're doing early morning cardio because your body will be completely cold — like giving a car a chance to warm up after it's been sitting in a garage overnight. Also, give your body time to rest between workouts. Get in a few hard workouts but then take one day off completely each week. For strength training, take at least one day off between sessions that work the same muscle group so you give the muscle fibers time to heal and strengthen. Finally, be sure you ask a trainer the proper form and technique for exercises and machines that are new to you to avoid pulling or straining a muscle.

> The best way to see your progress and maintain motivation is keeping track of the days you exercise in the 4-week journal in the back of this book. Seeing the days accumulate on your calendar will really keep you motivated for the times when the gym sounds less than tempting.

## Use your fitness journal!

In order to lose weight in a short amount of time, you need to expend more calories per day more than you eat. Therefore, exercise must become a part of your daily and weekly routine. The best way to see your progress and maintain motivation is keeping track of the days you exercise in the 4-week journal in the back of this book. Seeing the days accumulate on your calendar will really keep you motivated for the times when the gym sounds less than tempting. Write down the activity, the duration of time, reps, and the intensity (or weight, if strength training). Keep track of everything you do, and don't underestimate what may seem like a smaller activity, such as walking your dog. Consider that a 150-pound person will burn 100 calories from just a 20-minute walk at a moderate pace. Every little bit counts, just like with calories, so write it down and applaud yourself for making time throughout the day to get moving.

## Join an online weight-loss community

Create a profile page at an online weight-loss and fitness community and you'll have instant access to a huge group of people with similar goals, questions, obstacles, and tips for success. Seeing what works for others gives you motivation, and hearing about the ups and downs of exercise and losing weight from real people provides comfort and a sense of solidarity.

> Consider a virtual trainer — a real person who will create a fitness plan specifically for you based on your goals and the equipment you have available. You'll get online tutorials, text message reminders, and email check-ins from your trainer.

### Enlist a virtual trainer

Hiring a personal trainer can be a great motivator and learning experience, but not everyone is ready for the time or money commitment it requires. A terrific option is a virtual trainer. A real person will create a fitness plan specifically for you based on your goals and the equipment you have available. You'll get online tutorials on the proper form for exercises, worksheets for tracking progress, and accountability in the form of reminders and check-ins from your virtual trainer.

## Never give up!

"Don't give up, don't ever give up," legendary college basketball coach Jim Valvano told the crowd at the 1993 ESPY Awards, a night to celebrate the accomplishments of the greatest athletes in the world. Inspired by Valvano's fight against bone cancer, the athletes in the room also knew plenty about the resilience it takes to stay in top shape and perform under the most pressure imaginable. Valvano's words should inspire you, too!

Losing weight is a journey that takes determination and resilience, and exercise can be struggle if you haven't always been active. If you have had a busy day of work or family, it is tempting to spend an evening on the couch instead of going for a run or bike ride. One of the toughest things is getting back on an exercise schedule after you've missed a few days. But don't decide you've failed. If you skip a day of your workout, tell yourself you'll start again tomorrow. If you overindulge at a meal, be firm that you will have a longer, tougher workout the next day. If you feel like skipping the gym, tell yourself you'll do 30 minutes (odds are, you'll stay longer). Don't give up!

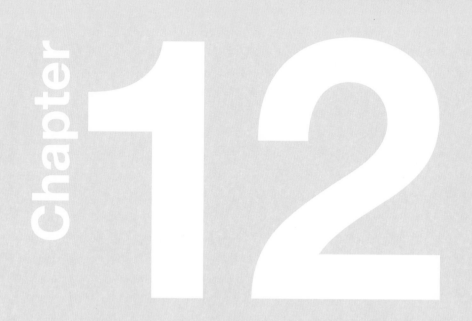

# Chapter 12

"Without discipline, there's no life at all."

~ Katharine Hepburn

# Maximizing Your Workouts

**To lose up to 10 pounds in a short amount of time** you need to make the most of every workout or physical activity you perform. You don't want to do the same exercises or routine every day for weeks. To optimize the amount of calories and body fat you burn during each workout and lose as much weight as you can, use the tips and tricks in this chapter to learn: when and how to work out; how to dress for your chosen activity; and how to stay motivated on days when you're feeling sluggish or lazy.

There is a lot to learn and remember when starting an intense fitness program like this one. In this chapter, you'll learn the right amount of weight you should be lifting during strength training, how to calculate your maximum and target heart rates, find how much water you should be drinking, and determine the best time to get new shoes as well as which type to buy.

Use the tips, formulas, and principles of fitness in this chapter to maximize your workout results. Nothing will make you feel better or more excited to maintain your program. With just a few weeks to go to lose weight, you have no time to waste!

### Work the "afterburn"

Do cardiovascular exercise first thing in the morning! During the night, your body becomes depleted of your primary energy source, carbohydrates. With that in short supply, your body begins to work from its secondary source, which is body fat. During a pre-breakfast morning workout, the body will burn more fat. You'll also have what is called the "afterburn effect," which means that metabolism stays elevated for several hours after your workout. Finally, working out in the morning gives you an endorphin rush and energy boost. This natural high can last for hours — even better than coffee!

### Lift the right amount of weight

Building muscle helps you lose fat and drop unwanted pounds, but do you know how much is the right amount of weight to lift during strength training? If you lift weights that are too light, you won't see improvements in strength or muscle tone. If you lift weights that are too heavy, you'll compromise form and risk getting injured. You want to be able to perform 8 to 12 repetitions per set, choosing weights heavy enough that you struggle through your final few reps, but not so heavy that you sacrifice form. You should be maxed out by the last rep; if you feel like you could do another, increase the weight by 5 to 10 percent.

Another way to determine the weight you should be lifting is to find your "1 rep max" for an exercise (the weight at which you can only do 1 rep), then lift 60 to 80 percent of that amount.

## Know how and when to eat to maximize your workouts

It's important to know which foods to eat before and after you exercise. Carbs that are low in fat give you the energy you need to have a great workout. Protein helps with muscle repair and growth. Fat also acts as fuel for workouts, although you should eat mostly unsaturated fats, such as those from nuts, avocados, and fish.

Give yourself plenty of time for your body to digest a meal before working out, and specifically avoid fatty foods before exercising. Fats remain in your stomach longer, causing you to feel uncomfortable. However, having low blood sugar before a workout can cause dizziness and lethargy, so if you're famished, a small snack of peanut butter or low-fat cheese on whole wheat crackers can give you the boost you need to make it through an exercise session. After your workout, eating a meal packed with protein and carbohydrates within 2 hours can help replace energy-fueling glycogen stores.

During a pre-breakfast morning workout, the body will burn more fat. You'll also have what is called the "afterburn effect," which means that metabolism stays elevated for several hours after your workout.

## Include interval training to torch calories and body fat

Your mission is to reduce your caloric intake or burn more calories through exercise than you take in a day. Interval training is a great way to blast through

*Wearing the appropriate shoes for the activity you choose — from running to weight lifting to basketball — protects you from soreness and injury.*

calories and body fat because it combines short bursts of intense activity with periods of lighter activity. As your cardiovascular fitness improves, you'll be able to go longer and up the intensity of the more difficult portions, helping you burn even more calories.

Here is one interval training workout that burns 500 or more calories in an hour on a treadmill. Eventually, aim for a sprinting pace of at least 7.5 mph, a running pace of at least 6.0 mph, and a jogging pace of at least 5.0 mph. Begin at 0:00 on the treadmill and follow this 60-minute plan:

| | |
|---|---|
| 0:00–10:00 | Warm up jog |
| 10:00–10:20 | Sprint |
| 10:20–11:20 | Jog |
| 11:20–11:40 | Sprint |
| 11:40–12:40 | Jog |
| 12:40–13:00 | Sprint |
| 13:00–17:00 | Jog |
| 17:00–27:00 | Run |
| 27:00–31:00 | Jog |
| 31:00–35:00 | Run |
| 35:00–39:00 | Jog |
| 39:00–43:00 | Run |
| 43:00–47:00 | Jog |
| 47:00–51:00 | Run |
| 51:00–55:00 | Jog |
| 55:00–60:00 | Gradually slow pace to jog/walk to cool down |

## Wear the right shoes

Just like getting new exercise clothes, having the right shoes improves your workout. Wearing the appropriate shoes for the activity — from running to weight lifting to basketball — also protects you from soreness and injury. For instance, running shoes are designed for forward heel-to-toe motion and do not provide the right ankle support for the side-to-side motion of activities like kickboxing or step aerobics. And not all running shoes provide the same cushioning and support. For instance, depending on whether you supinate (run on the outside of your feet) or overpronate (your feet roll inward as you run), you will need different types of running shoes. If you check out your old shoes, you should be able to see where the heel is worn down. Or visit a specialty store to have your foot measured and your shoes professionally fit. A shoe should be snug but not be so tight that it puts pressure on the top of your foot or crushes your toes. And be sure to replace shoes every 300 to 500 miles, which you can monitor in your fitness journal.

## Stay hydrated

Proper hydration is one of the easiest and most effective ways of boosting workout performance. Water is necessary

### Did You Know?

Taking up long-distance running, cycling or swimming? Water is always a great choice for hydration and recovery, but what about the childhood favorite, chocolate milk? A study published in the *International Journal of Sport Nutrition and Exercise Metabolism* compared cyclists who consumed chocolate milk post-workout and found they performed just as well, if not better, than those who drank other sports drinks during the next cycling session. Chocolate milk has high water content for hydrating the body, but also has twice as much carbs and protein for replenishing tired muscles, as well as calcium, which the other drinks lack.

in order for metabolism to take place, so being properly hydrated helps your body turn food into the energy you need for exercising. Water also helps your body regulate its temperature through sweating. Because vigorous exercise causes you to lose large amounts of water through sweating, it is important to drink water before, during, and after each workout session. Drink between 8 and 16 ounces of water in the hour prior to working out. Replenish fluids by drinking 4 to 8 ounces of water every 15 minutes during your workout. During vigorous cardiovascular training, or if you're exercising in hot temperatures, increase your water consumption in order to replace water lost from sweating. Then drink between 8 and 16 ounces of water within 30 minutes of completing your exercise routine. Your muscles need water in order to recover from the stress of a workout. Drinking the correct amounts of water after your workout will help reduce muscle soreness and help you feel less tired.

> Build 1 or 2 "light days" into your weekly workout schedule, but make them count! Light days might include biking, walking, dynamic stretching (walking lunges, trunk twists, or arm circles, for instance), and swimming.

## Hydrate right!

It's extremely important to stay fully hydrated before, during, and after your workout — just don't reach for a sports drink that is full of unwanted calories. While slews of TV commercials featuring famous pro athletes lead you to believe that sports drinks like Gatorade and Vitamin Water help you stay fit and healthy, these drinks actually contain up to 200 calories and 35 grams of carbs per bottle. The promise that these drinks will give you the energy and electrolytes you need to have a great workout is really just a marketing ploy. For instance, Gatorade was originally developed to help college football players avoid dehydration and cramping during a rigorous training program in the humid summer months. A normal person like you, who is exercising at a much more moderate level, has no need for the carbs and calories in a sports drink. Water is always your best option. If you like the flavoring in sports drinks, try a low or no-calorie version, like Powerade Zero or Gatorade's G2.

## Don't overtrain

Want in on a fitness secret? There is such a thing as too much exercise. Let's say you're preparing to run a 5k race, and you start running several miles every day. You'll quickly notice that after a couple of weeks of training hard daily, your body begins to feel fatigued more quickly. Your muscles ache and you feel tired after just a short distance. You may find that you feel sore and even have trouble sleeping at night. These are all symptoms of overtraining. In order to lose weight quickly, you will need to do some form of exercise each day; however, you shouldn't aim for a high-intensity cardio or weight-lifting session every day. It's not realistic or good for your body, which needs periods of rest and recovery. Build one or two "light days" into your weekly workout schedule, but make them count! Schedule the same amount of time for your workout as a normal day, just exercise at a lower intensity. Light days might include biking, walking, dynamic stretching (walking lunges, trunk twists, or arm circles, for instance), and swimming. Keep your body in motion but make sure you're giving hardworking muscle groups time to rest and recover, so you're full of energy and stamina for your next tough workout.

In addition to reps with weights; consider power yoga, which can burn more than 400 calories per hour, and works multiple muscle groups at once. Yoga is a great workout because you're lifting your own body weight in many poses.

## Work toward your target heart rate

If you're not working out within your target heart rate zone, you're not getting the maximum benefits. The "fat burning zone," which burns the most calories and body fat stores, is reached at about 60 to 70 percent of your maximum heart rate. To calculate your maximum heart rate, subtract your age from 226 for women, 220 for men. Then, multiply that number by 0.6 (60 percent) or 0.7 (70 percent) to find the number of beats per minute that is your target heart rate.

To determine whether you're in that zone during your workout, either wear a heart rate monitor or take your pulse for 10 seconds and multiply the number of beats by 6. Adjust your intensity depending on whether you are above or below your target heart rate.

As your level of fitness improves, you should up the intensity of your workouts. For example, when running, aim for a sprinting pace of at least 7.5 mph, a running pace of at least 6.0 mph, and a jogging pace of at least 5.0 mph.

## Exercise muscles in proper progression to maximize results.

When you're working a variety of muscles during a strength-training sequence, order is important. If your workout includes a variety of weight lifting exercises, begin with your larger muscle groups and move to the smaller muscles. This allows for optimal performance of the most demanding exercises when your fatigue levels are at their lowest, and you feel energized and fresh. The most important thing is to be sure that you have enough energy to complete your entire workout. It is better to do less and complete the entire circuit than to neglect a muscle group or do an uneven number of reps from one side of the body to the other.

## Variety is the spice of life

Variety helps keep you happy and motivated in both your diet and your workouts. If you restrict your diet to the point that you're eating only fish and salad, for instance, you'll quickly lose interest and enthusiasm.

Variety also keeps your weight loss and calorie burning from plateauing. If you do the same exercises at the same intensity day after day, working out will get boring and your body will stop burning fat and calories as quickly. You'll find your weight loss comes to a standstill. You need to plan for workouts that work different muscle groups at different intensities throughout the week. Because you're trying to torch through unwanted pounds, you'll want to focus on cardio but also complement it with strength training.

Carbs that are low in fat give you the energy you need to have a great workout. Protein helps with muscle repair and growth. Fat also acts as fuel for workouts, although you should eat mostly unsaturated fats.

In addition to reps with weights, consider power yoga, which can burn more than 400 calories per hour and works multiple muscle groups at once. Yoga is such a great workout because you're lifting your own body weight in many poses. Whatever you choose to do, creating a varied workout schedule is imperative to losing 10 pounds.

# Chapter 13

"Failure is not fatal, but failure to change might be."

~ John Wooden

# Ultimate Fitness Tips

You're well on your way to a successful diet and fitness program and, by now, you're seeing the weight drop off, feeling healthier, and enjoying more energy than ever. To continue making progress, you need to keep your body from plateauing and your dedication from waning.

To round out your program, you need a few powerful secrets. In this chapter, learn how to exercise efficiently, stay inspired, and breeze through physical activity on a daily basis, without your workout feeling like "work."

Motivation, seeing results, and enjoyment are the keys to sticking with a fitness plan for 4 weeks, or any amount of time. This book has given you all the tools you need to lose up to 10 pounds faster than you ever thought possible — use this final fitness chapter to rev up your workouts and get the very most from every minute of physical activity you do.

## Make a music playlist to stay motivated

Music has been proven to help people work out longer and with more energy, as well as providing a distraction from fatigue. Dr. Costas Karageorghis, who has studied the effects of music on physical performance for 20 years, says that a good workout song should be between 120 and 140 beats-per-minute, which corresponds to the average person's heart rate while performing moderate exercise (up the tempo if you're working out harder). Most pop, rap, heavy metal, and many rock songs fall into this tempo range. Even if it's not your favorite artist or a type of music that you'd listen to in your car, an upbeat song can help keep you going when your energy is low or you're nearing the end of a tough workout.

Work out with someone you see often, such as your neighbor, coworker, roommate or spouse, and you'll be best able to hold each other accountable.

## Invest in new workout clothes

When you feel confident and have the proper exercise clothes, you will be more motivated to exercise, and you'll work out longer too. Invest in a few new pieces of workout clothing and you'll be inspired and excited to wear them! Choose shirts, shorts, pants, and sports bras in breathable, quick-drying fabrics that wick sweat away from the body. Exercise clothes should also stretch and move with you. Finally, be sure to get what you need for the specific activities you'll be engaging in, such as compression shorts for biking, form-fitting pants for yoga, and supportive undergarments for running.

## Hydrate and replenish with coconut water

Coconut water is one of the purest natural liquids around, second only to real water. It's one of nature's best superfoods! Unlike sugary sports drinks, coconut water contains natural electrolytes for energy and hydration but with minimal calories (typically about 60 per bottle). Coconut water has no added sugar, and with more potassium than a banana and 15 times more than most sports drinks, it prevents cramping and promotes muscle recovery during and after a workout. It also has myriad weight-loss benefits, such as increasing metabolism and promoting healthy thyroid function.

You can buy individual servings of coconut water at most health food stores and at many gyms and fitness studios. Its natural properties and benefits to your health and exercise program make it a favorite of cyclists, runners, trainers, yogis, and more.

## Use plyometrics to blast calories

Plyometrics are a great way to burn calories in a short amount of time. These types of exercise are designed to produce fast, powerful movements. The muscle is loaded and then contracted in a rapid sequence. When these exercises are done in succession they burn calories quickly. Plyometrics are great because they are strength-building exercises that require endurance and cardiovascular stamina.

You can try mixing jump rope, jumping jacks, squat jumps, box jumps, and other plyometric activities into your normal workouts.

## Get Netflix

No one is recommending you sit on your couch with movies all night —
but Netflix is actually a great, inexpensive way to work out at home! Their
wide selection of exercise and fitness DVDs includes dance, aerobics, yoga,
Pilates, strength training, and more. Some DVDs are available for rental,
delivered right to your mailbox, and can be kept as long as you like, and others
can be watched instantly online or on a gaming console like Wii or Xbox.
Workout DVDs are perfect for the times when you need a quick, 30-minute blast,
don't have time to drive to the gym, or want to try something new in the
privacy of your living room. Or maybe you're not sure if Hollywood trainer
Jillian Michaels' *30-Day Shred* is right for you? Netflix gives you the option to
try specific exercise DVDs before buying them. Just be sure to type in the name of
the video you want into the Search bar — the "Browse" feature shows only a
very limited number of choices.

> ## Did You Know?
> According to a *Men's Fitness* magazine survey of more than 5,000 readers, guys' favorite part of a woman's body is her butt (40 percent), beating out legs and even breasts! Guys preferred voluptuous bodies, like Kim Kardashian's, and athletic bodies, like Cameron Diaz's over thin stick-figures. All the more motivation to define curves and build sexy muscles.

### Find a fitness buddy

Losing weight and getting active are always easier with a partner, so invite
a spouse or friend to join you in your weight-loss efforts, especially if he
or she seems threatened by or uncomfortable with your weight loss. The
great things about a workout buddy is he or she keeps you accountable,
motivated on the days when you don't feel like exercising, and keeps you
company on hikes, bike rides, and rock climbing trips. Plus, if you're just
trying out a new form of exercise, such as surfing or kickboxing, having a

partner can make it more fun and less scary. Make your workout buddy someone you see often, such as your neighbor, coworker, roommate or spouse, and you'll be best able to hold each other accountable. You'll also have someone to celebrate with when you both drop 10 pounds!

A good workout song should be between 120 and 140 beats-per-minute, which corresponds to the average person's heart rate while exercising.

### Schedule a cardio session around a TV show or sporting event

Running or bicycling for an hour or more in a gym can get dull fast. One tip for getting through a longer cardio session is to plan it for a time when a favorite show, movie, or sporting event is on TV. Time will fly by when you're watching the Lakers game or an hour-long sitcom. Just be sure to do this when you have at least 45 minutes or more of cardio and you can work at a steady pace and zone out a bit. You won't want to be distracted by the TV screen if you're trying to get through 30 minutes of interval training, for instance.

### Get a boost from pre-workout caffeine

The caffeine in natural sources such as coffee, green tea, or in pill form, benefits your workouts because it acts as a thermogenic. Themorgenics speed up your body's functions, including breath and heart rate, encouraging the body to use calories more quickly. Don't overdo it when it comes to caffeine, of course. Listen to your body, and if you feel light-headed, dizzy or faint, stop what you're doing immediately, rest for a few minutes, and abstain from caffeine in the future. Otherwise, unless you're exercising at high altitudes, suffer from high blood pressure, or another heart condition, taking 100 to 200 mg (one cup of coffee has about 100 mg) of caffeine 45 minutes before a workout can help you burn fat stores, speed up your metabolism, and help you power through a workout.

## Count your steps with a pedometer

Start wearing a pedometer daily to measure how many steps you're taking and how many calories you're burning. Pedometers clip to your belt or pocket — or any spot where they will be perpendicular to the ground. They come in a variety of styles and price points — for less than $20 you can get a sleek, simple device that counts steps and calculates calories burned. Deluxe models play music, have audio features, and allow you to upload your daily stats into your computer to track your progress and meet goals. Many new mp3 players come with built-in pedometers as well. You'll want to reference consumer reports that test the efficiency and accuracy of different makes and models.

Drinking several cups of green tea can boost your workout and burns about 70 extra calories per day.

For $99, a new Microsoft product called Fitbit accurately tracks your calories burned, steps taken, distance traveled, and even sleep quality. On your Fitbit profile, you enter the calories you ate for the day, and the data from your Fitbit device automatically calculates if you've met the distance and calorie goals you set for the day and week.

## Blow off the gym!

Many people enjoy the routine schedule of going to the same location every day, but others find the gym stifling and somewhat limiting. Or you may feel lost among the confusing machines, bustling trainers, and intense gym rats. Be it burnout or pure intimidation, you may be looking for an alternative to the gym.

Naturally, getting outside in the fresh air is your best choice. If you live in a city where weather permits, add a fun activity to your weekly workout schedule — bike rides, hiking, surfing, horseback riding, rock climbing. Try something new to shake things up and stay motivated. Boot camps are also a great way to burn hundreds of calories in a short amount of time. Beach or park boot camps are popping up all over the country, as well as indoor sessions that combine strength training with cardio. Boot camps use interval training — bursts of activity with short rests in between exercises — to blast calories and fat. Another gym alternative is joining a private yoga or Pilates studio. You'll get focused, professional instructors and classes without the overwhelming nature of a gym atmosphere.

Caffeine benefits your workouts because it acts as a thermogenic. Themorgenics speed up your body's functions, including breath and heart rate, encouraging the body to use calories more quickly.

There are really hundreds of exercises, classes, and groups available. Check out the website MeetUp.com to find out what's going on in your area. From surfing moms to salsa dancing clubs, if you can imagine it, it's out there.

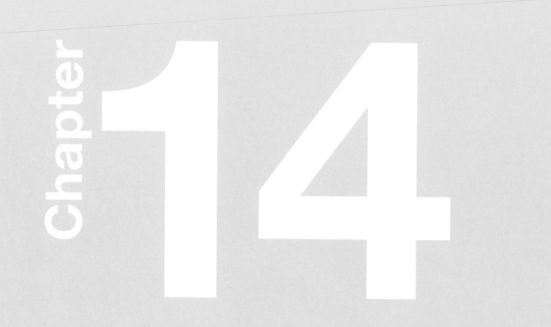

# Chapter 14

"It's not who you are that holds you back, it's who you think you're not."

~ Unknown

# Activities & Calories Burned

**All types of physical activity burn calories.** You don't have to slave away at a gym — normal daily activities, chores, and errands also require your body to burn calories in addition to exercise.

This chapter highlights some of the typical physical activities, from sports to household chores, that you can do to burn calories while losing 10 pounds. They range from light to moderate to vigorous, so incorporate something from each list every day or combine activities.

Be aware that the exact number of calories you will burn for each activity varies based on your weight. The following list is an approximation for someone who weighs 150 pounds. If you weigh more, you will burn slightly more calories; if you weigh less than 150 pounds, you will burn slightly fewer calories. If you require an exact count, there are many websites that can estimate calories burned based on your weight, intensity of the workout, and the length of time you exercised.

## Light Activities: 150 or Less Cal/Hr.

Billiards. . . . . . . . . . . . . . . . . . . . . . . . . . . . . . . . . . . . . . . . . . . . . .140

Lying down/sleeping . . . . . . . . . . . . . . . . . . . . . . . . . . . . . . . . .60

Office work. . . . . . . . . . . . . . . . . . . . . . . . . . . . . . . . . . . . . .140

Sitting . . . . . . . . . . . . . . . . . . . . . . . . . . . . . . . . . . . . . . . . .80

Standing . . . . . . . . . . . . . . . . . . . . . . . . . . . . . . . . . . . . . . . .100

## Moderate Activities: 150-350 Cal/Hr.

Aerobic dancing . . . . . . . . . . . . . . . . . . . . . . . . . . . . . . . . . .340

Ballroom dancing . . . . . . . . . . . . . . . . . . . . . . . . . . . . . . . . .210

Bicycling (5 mph) . . . . . . . . . . . . . . . . . . . . . . . . . . . . . . . . .170

Bowling. . . . . . . . . . . . . . . . . . . . . . . . . . . . . . . . . . . . . . . .160

Canoeing (2.5 mph) . . . . . . . . . . . . . . . . . . . . . . . . . . . . . . .170

Dancing (social) . . . . . . . . . . . . . . . . . . . . . . . . . . . . . . . . . .210

Gardening (moderate). . . . . . . . . . . . . . . . . . . . . . . . . . . . . .270

Golf (with cart). . . . . . . . . . . . . . . . . . . . . . . . . . . . . . . . . . .180

Golf (without cart) . . . . . . . . . . . . . . . . . . . . . . . . . . . . . . . .320

Grocery shopping . . . . . . . . . . . . . . . . . . . . . . . . . . . . . . . . .180

Horseback riding (sitting trot). . . . . . . . . . . . . . . . . . . . . . . .250

Light housework/cleaning, etc. . . . . . . . . . . . . . . . . . . . . . . .250

Pilates . . . . . . . . . . . . . . . . . . . . . . . . . . . . . . . . . . . . . . . . .240

Ping-pong . . . . . . . . . . . . . . . . . . . . . . . . . . . . . . . . . . . . . .270

Surfing . . . . . . . . . . . . . . . . . . . . . . . . . . . . . . . . . . . . . . . .300

Swimming (20 yards/min). . . . . . . . . . . . . . . . . . . . . . . . . .290

Tennis (recreational doubles). . . . . . . . . . . . . . . . . . . . . . . .310

Vacuuming . . . . . . . . . . . . . . . . . . . . . . . . . . . . . . . . . . . . .220

Volleyball (recreational) . . . . . . . . . . . . . . . . . . . . . . . . . . . .260

Walking (2 mph). . . . . . . . . . . . . . . . . . . . . . . . . . . . . . . . .200

Walking (3 mph) . . . . . . . . . . . . . . . . . . . . . . . . . . . . . . . . .240

Walking (4 mph). . . . . . . . . . . . . . . . . . . . . . . . . . . . . . . . .300

## Vigorous Activities: 350 or More Cal/Hr.

Aerobics (step). . . . . . . . . . . . . . . . . . . . . . . . . . . . . . . . . . . .440

Backpacking (10 lb load). . . . . . . . . . . . . . . . . . . . . . . . . . . .540

Badminton . . . . . . . . . . . . . . . . . . . . . . . . . . . . . . . . . . . . . . .450

Basketball (competitive) . . . . . . . . . . . . . . . . . . . . . . . . . . .660

Basketball (leisure) . . . . . . . . . . . . . . . . . . . . . . . . . . . . . . .390

Bicycling (10 mph). . . . . . . . . . . . . . . . . . . . . . . . . . . . . . . .375

Bicycling (13 mph) . . . . . . . . . . . . . . . . . . . . . . . . . . . . . . . .600

Cross country skiing (leisurely). . . . . . . . . . . . . . . . . . . . . .460

Cross country skiing (moderate) . . . . . . . . . . . . . . . . . . . . .660

Hiking . . . . . . . . . . . . . . . . . . . . . . . . . . . . . . . . . . . . . . . . . .460

Ice skating (9 mph) . . . . . . . . . . . . . . . . . . . . . . . . . . . . . . .384

Jogging (5 mph). . . . . . . . . . . . . . . . . . . . . . . . . . . . . . . . . .550

Jogging (6 mph) . . . . . . . . . . . . . . . . . . . . . . . . . . . . . . . . . .690

Racquetball. . . . . . . . . . . . . . . . . . . . . . . . . . . . . . . . . . . . . .620

Rock Climbing . . . . . . . . . . . . . . . . . . . . . . . . . . . . . . . . . . .740

Rollerblading . . . . . . . . . . . . . . . . . . . . . . . . . . . . . . . . . . . .384

Rowing machine . . . . . . . . . . . . . . . . . . . . . . . . . . . . . . . . . .540

Running (8 mph). . . . . . . . . . . . . . . . . . . . . . . . . . . . . . . . . .900

Scuba diving . . . . . . . . . . . . . . . . . . . . . . . . . . . . . . . . . . . . .570

Shoveling snow . . . . . . . . . . . . . . . . . . . . . . . . . . . . . . . . . . .580

Soccer . . . . . . . . . . . . . . . . . . . . . . . . . . . . . . . . . . . . . . . . . .580

Spinning . . . . . . . . . . . . . . . . . . . . . . . . . . . . . . . . . . . . . . . .650

Stair climber machine . . . . . . . . . . . . . . . . . . . . . . . . . . . . .480

Swimming (50 yards/min.) . . . . . . . . . . . . . . . . . . . . . . . . . .680

Water aerobics. . . . . . . . . . . . . . . . . . . . . . . . . . . . . . . . . . .400

Water skiing . . . . . . . . . . . . . . . . . . . . . . . . . . . . . . . . . . . . .480

Weight training (30 sec. between sets). . . . . . . . . . . . . . . . .760

Weight training (60 sec. between sets). . . . . . . . . . . . . . . . .570

Yoga (power). . . . . . . . . . . . . . . . . . . . . . . . . . . . . . . . . . . . .400

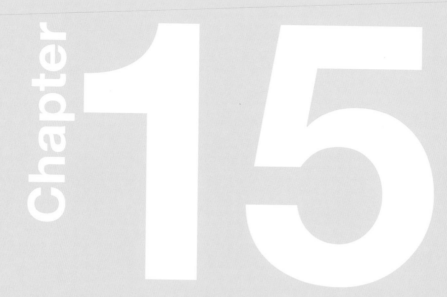

Chapter

# 15

"The greatest wealth is health."

~ Virgil

# Lose Weight Fast Diet
# Exercise Plan

**Losing weight fast requires a fitness plan full of** high-intensity, calorie-blasting exercises that work the whole body. *The Lose Weight Fast Diet* Exercise Plan is designed to target multiple muscle groups, build core strength, and elevate the heart rate to burn body fat.

6 days out of each week you will pair a strength training circuit with a cardio circuit. You'll need water, stable exercise shoes, and moveable, breathable workout clothing. Each day, you will do 1 of 2 core strength training sets, an upper body circuit, or a lower body circuit. For cardio, you can choose from a custom walking or running circuit or choose your own activity. The seventh day of the week is to rest and recuperate.

Every strength training exercise comes with step-by-step instructions, as well as modifications to make the move easier or harder. You may want to challenge yourself more on some exercises, or modify some moves to avoid injury or account for soreness.

For the cardio circuits, you will be able to work faster and harder as your fitness level improves.

## How to Do the Exercise Plan

You will need to set aside about 60 minutes to complete this workout plan. Do each exercise for 50 seconds, as many reps as you can do in that time without sacrificing form. Take a 10-second rest to get ready for the next exercise. Keep your eye on a stopwatch, timer on an mp3 player, or clock with a seconds hand. Complete all 6 exercises in the strength training circuit, then repeat the full circuit for a second round, and again for a third. After you have completed 3 rounds of the strength training circuit, take a 2-minute water break and move on to the cardio circuit. Do the same for the cardio circuit.

## Warming Up and Cooling Down

Always begin and end your strength training and cardio workouts with a 5 to 10-minute warm-up and cool-down. Walk, lightly jog, or run in place to loosen the muscles. Next, stretch to prepare your muscles for work and prevent injury.

Important stretches include holding the heel close to the glute to stretch the quad muscle, reaching toward the toes to stretch hamstrings, calf stretches against a wall, and stretching your arms behind your head and across the chest to loosen shoulders, chest, biceps and triceps.

The same routine after your workout will bring the heart rate down, help the body recover, and prevent soreness.

## Your Workout Schedule

You only have 2 short weeks to get the body you've always wanted, so work hard and push yourself, even if it's to do one more rep! You'll love the feeling of success and pride you'll get after a tough workout. The body, strength, and shape you've always wanted is just a couple of weeks away.

## Notes:

# Core 1

**Equipment:**
Stability ball
Dumbbells

Strength training is a very important part of losing weight. The following workout will lengthen and tone your core while replacing body fat with muscle, which burns three times as many calories as fat.

The exercises in this section work all parts of the core, including the abs, obliques, and lower back. You'll also work the arms, shoulders, and more. When coupled with a cardio program, these moves will help you get in shape quickly. Plus, they're fun and challenging!

# Scorpion Plank

1. Start in plank position with hands under shoulders. Pull the right knee toward the left elbow and twist your torso to the left.

2. Return to starting position and switch sides, twisting the other side with the left leg. Keep your core engaged and don't let your hips sag.

**Make it easier:** Bring the knee in to the chest and skip the twist.

**Make it harder:** Place your feet up on a stability ball to force the core to work even harder.

# Crunch on Stability Ball

1. Start with your shoulders, lower back, and hips on a stability ball. Interlace your fingers behind your head, and pull your belly button in toward your spine.

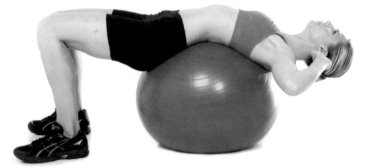

2. Raise your head and shoulders in a crunch, pausing at the top and returning slowly to a start position.

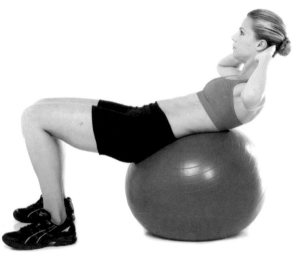

Make it easier: Crunch on the ground without the stability ball.

Make it harder: Hold a dumbbell in both hands as you crunch.

# Superman Roll

1. Lie flat on your stomach with your arms straight out in front of you and legs straight out behind you, both about shoulder-width apart. Lift your legs and arms simultaneously at least 6 inches off the ground.

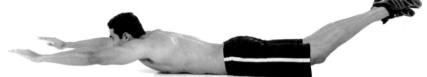

2. In a fluid motion, roll over onto your back, keeping your arms and legs elevated off the ground and engaging the core. Reach your arms and legs away from the body, lengthening the core.

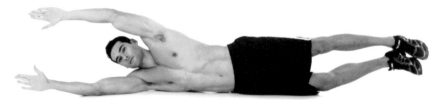

3. Continue to roll back and forth, pausing after each roll until you need to rest.

Make it easier: Lift only your arms or only your legs instead of both at the same time.

Make it harder: Add a crunch when you are on your back.

# Side Plank with Push-up

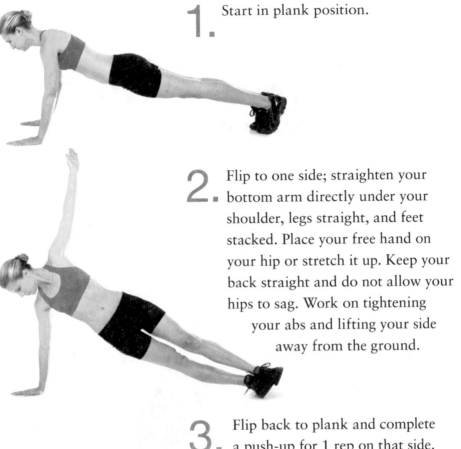

**1.** Start in plank position.

**2.** Flip to one side; straighten your bottom arm directly under your shoulder, legs straight, and feet stacked. Place your free hand on your hip or stretch it up. Keep your back straight and do not allow your hips to sag. Work on tightening your abs and lifting your side away from the ground.

**3.** Flip back to plank and complete a push-up for 1 rep on that side. Repeat, switching sides.

Make it easier: Place one knee on the ground. Skip the push-up.

Make it harder: Lift the top leg up 6 inches.

# V-Up

1. Lie on the floor with arms stretched above the head and legs out straight out in front.

2. Simultaneously, lift your chest and the legs straight up, reaching the fingers toward the toes. Lower back to the ground for 1 rep.

Make it easier: Bend your knees and pull them in to the chest, keeping your arms parallel to the floor.

Make it harder : Hold a weight in your hands as you reach for your toes.

# Russian Twist with Dumbbell

1. Sit upright with your legs bent and feet on the floor. Hold arms out in front of you and hold a dumbbell with both hands. Lean slightly back so your upper body forms a 45-degree angle with the floor.

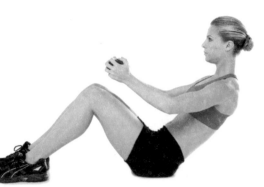

2. Rotate your arms and the dumbbell as far to one side as you can, reaching down while you squeeze your abs and obliques.

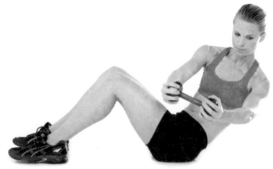

3. Return to center and twist to the other side. Rotate from your core, not your hips.

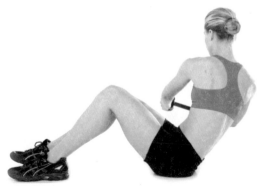

Make it easier: Don't use a dumbbell.

Make it harder: Lift your feet off the floor and don't let them touch at any time.

## Notes:

# Core 2

**Equipment:**
Dumbbells

This second set of core exercises will whip your middle into shape in just 30 days. You'll feel leaner and stronger, especially when you combine these moves with a cardio program.

Don't forget to challenge yourself as much as possible, and modify as necessary to push yourself or account for injuries or sore muscles.

# Hip Crossover with Stability Ball

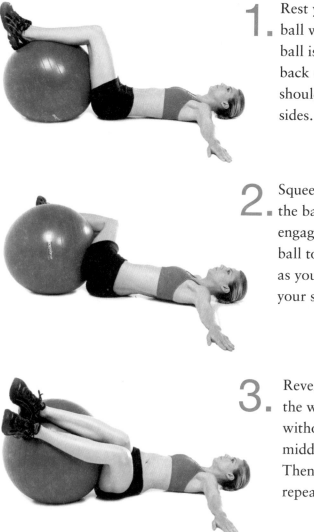

1. Rest your feet on a stability ball with knees bent, so the ball is resting against the back of the thighs. Arms should be straight out to the sides.

2. Squeezing the ball against the backs of the thighs and engaging the core, drop the ball to the right side, as low as you can without lifting your shoulders off the floor.

3. Reverse the movement all the way to the left side, without pausing in the middle, to complete 1 rep. Then return to center and repeat.

Make it easier: Don't lower yourself as close to the ground.

Make it harder: Move slowly and with control.

# Jackknife & Push-up on Stability Ball

**1.** Begin in a plank position with your hands under your shoulders and the tops of the feet and shins elevated on a stability ball.

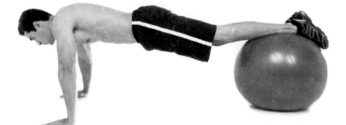

**2.** Without rounding the lower back, bend your knees and use your core muscles to pull the ball in toward the body.

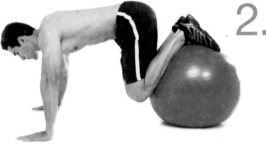

**3.** Push the ball back out to plank, then lower into a push-up to complete 1 rep.

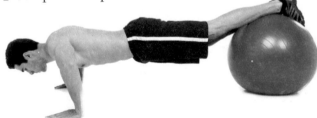

Make it easier: Skip the push-up.

Make it harder: Instead of bending your knees, keep the legs straight and lift your hips up so you end up in a pike position.

# Beetle Crunch

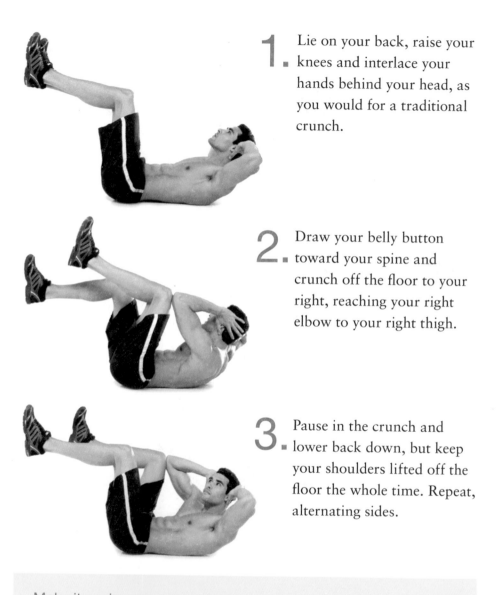

1. Lie on your back, raise your knees and interlace your hands behind your head, as you would for a traditional crunch.

2. Draw your belly button toward your spine and crunch off the floor to your right, reaching your right elbow to your right thigh.

3. Pause in the crunch and lower back down, but keep your shoulders lifted off the floor the whole time. Repeat, alternating sides.

Make it easier: Allow the upper back and shoulders to rest on the ground between reps.

Make it harder : Touch your elbow to both knees, instead of only one.

# X Sit-ups

1. Lie on your back with arms and legs stretched out, slightly wider than shoulder-width apart, forming an X-shape. Then, fold your left hand behind your head.

2. Sit straight up, pointing your right hand up above the head as if you are reaching for the ceiling.

3. Next, crunch forward, reaching the right hand across the body to touch the left toe.

Reverse the movement and lie back down for 1 rep. Switch arms and repeat on the opposite side.

Make it easier: Point both hands out in front of you and crunch with this modified arm position.

Make it harder: Sit cross-legged to force the core to work harder. Engage the core and don't let your lower back hunch over.

# Bicycles

1. Lie on your back with your knees bent at a 90-degree angle.

2. Lace your fingers behind your head. Lift your head and shoulders, exhale and twist to one side, bringing your knee in to touch your opposite elbow, while straightening the other leg. Return to center, inhale.

3. Exhale and twist to the opposite side.

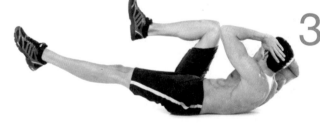

Make it easier: Keep feet on the ground and slide heels along the floor using a towel.

Make it harder: Perform bicycles as fast as you can, making sure to rotate from the core.

# Roll-out on Stability Ball

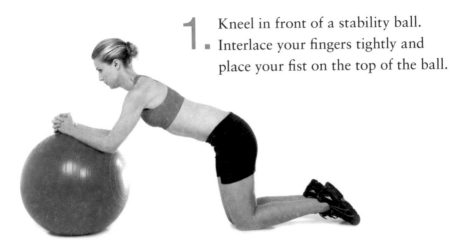

1. Kneel in front of a stability ball. Interlace your fingers tightly and place your fist on the top of the ball.

2. Keeping your core engaged, slowly roll the ball out and away from you, straightening your arms as much as you can without sagging your hips or collapsing through the lower back. Use your abs to pull you back to the starting position.

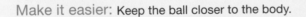

Make it easier: Keep the ball closer to the body.

Make it harder: Push the ball out further and keep the ball under your wrists.

## Notes:

# Upper Body

These upper body exercises will work different parts of your chest, back, shoulders, as well as upper and lower arms.

Challenge yourself, but don't sacrifice form. It's better to do fewer high-quality reps than a higher number of reps with bad form.

# Judo Push-ups

1. Put your hands and feet flat on the ground with your hips lifted so your body forms an inverted V shape.

2. Keeping your hips up, bend your arms out to the side, and lower your upper body until your chin is near the floor.

3. Lower your hips toward the floor while you lift your upper body simultaneously. Then slide back into the original position, reversing the way you went in for 1 rep.

Make it easier: Put your knees on the ground as your lower your hips to the floor.

Make it harder : Lift one leg.

# Chest Fly on Stability Ball

1. Lie in a table position with your shoulders and upper back on a stability ball and feet on the floor, hip-width apart. Hold a dumbbell in each hand, above your chest, palms facing out. Keep your core engaged and your hips lifted.

2. With slightly bent elbows, lower your arms down and back. Don't let arms go below chest-height. Press arms back up and touch them to complete 1 rep.

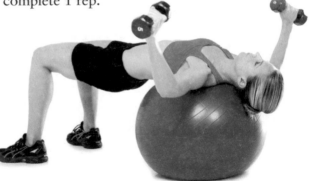

Make it easier: Use lighter weights.

Make it harder: Use heavier weights, but don't sacrifice form.

# Bent Row

**1.** Stand with feet shoulder-width apart, holding a dumbbell in each hand, palms facing your thighs. Hinge forward at the hips so your torso is parallel or almost parallel to the floor.

**2.** Bend at the elbows, pulling arms straight back until weights are at chest-height. Squeeze the shoulder blades at the top of the row; then lower your arms for 1 rep.

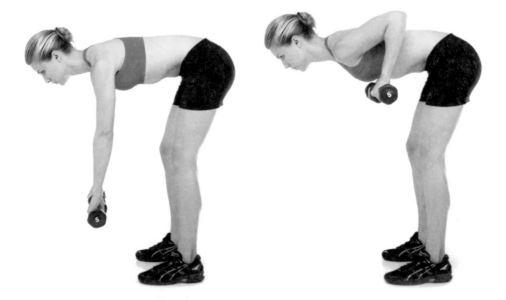

Make it easier: Use a lighter weight.

Make it harder: Extend one leg behind you into an arabesque as you hinge forward, forming a T with your body. You will use your abs and glutes to maintain balance.

# Tricep Kickbacks

1. Stand with feet shoulder-width apart, holding a dumbbell in each hand, palms facing your sides. Hinge forward at the hips so your torso is parallel, or almost parallel to the floor.

2. Bend at the elbow in a 45-degree angle and pull up your right arm so the upper arm is parallel to the floor.

3. Keeping your right upper arm still, raise your forearm so the weight stretches out behind you and your arm is straight, squeezing the tricep and upper back. Reverse the motion for 1 rep. Repeat as many times as you can, switching arms at the 25-second mark.

Make it easier: Use a lighter weight.

Make it harder: Extend both arms at the same time, which requires more back stabilization and makes you perform twice as many reps.

# Dumbbell Swing

**1.** Hold a dumbbell with an overhand grip (palm facing toward the body) between your legs; bend your knees and squat down.

**2.** Thrusting through your glutes and hips, and squeezing the shoulders, stand up and swing the dumbbell up until it is chest-high.

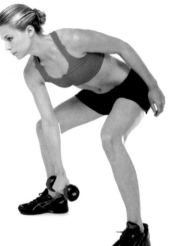

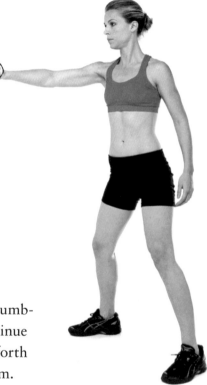

**3.** Squat back down and swing the dumbbell back between your legs. Continue swinging the dumbbell back and forth fluidly and without sacrificing form. Switch arms at the 25-second mark.

Make it easier: Hold the dumbbell with two hands.

Make it harder: Use a heavier weight but don't sacrifice form.

# Mountain Climbers

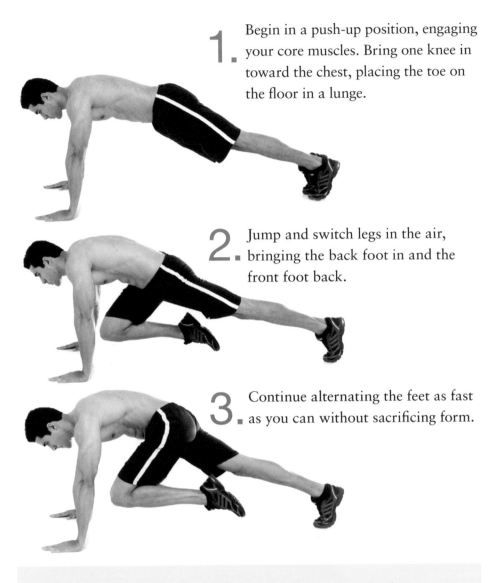

**1.** Begin in a push-up position, engaging your core muscles. Bring one knee in toward the chest, placing the toe on the floor in a lunge.

**2.** Jump and switch legs in the air, bringing the back foot in and the front foot back.

**3.** Continue alternating the feet as fast as you can without sacrificing form.

Make it easier: If you're not familiar with this exercise, go slowly and focus on switching your legs in and out of the low lunge. You can "walk" through this exercise until you feel comfortable with the motion.

Make it harder: Go faster without letting the knees bow out.

# Weed Puller

**1.** Bend forward at the waist so your torso forms nearly a 45-degree angle with the floor. Hold one dumbbell in your right hand, palm facing in, and your arm straight down.

**2.** Pull the dumbbell up toward your chest and rotate out to the right side, twisting your torso up (imagine pulling a weed out of the ground). Lower back to the starting position and repeat, switching the dumbbell to the other hand at the 25-second mark.

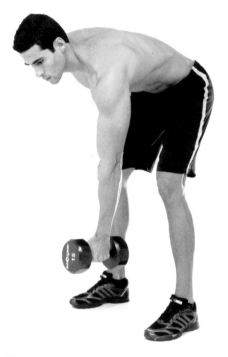

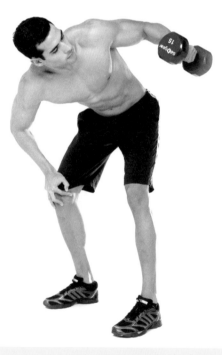

Make it easier: Use a lighter weight.

Make it harder : Use a heavier weight.

# Lower Body

**Equipment:**
Stability ball
Dumbbells

This series of lunges, raises, and plyometric moves will whip your thighs, hamstrings, glutes, and calves into shape in no time! You'll feel stronger and more explosive throughout the entire lower body.

A lower body circuit combined with cardio work can be a lot on the legs, so be sure to walk for a few minutes or jog in place to warm up the body completely. And remember, concentrate on using proper form to make the most of these moves.

# Side Lunge with Chop

**1.** Stand with legs shoulder-width apart and toes slightly turned out, holding a dumbbell on both ends at chest-height.

**2.** Lunge out to the right side and bring the dumbbell across the front of the body and down toward the outer edge of the foot.

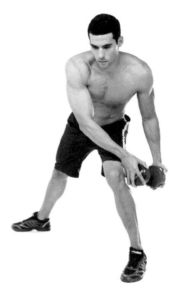

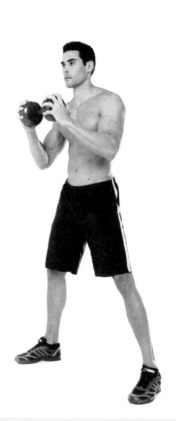

**3.** Press back up through the foot and thigh to return to a standing position. Repeat until the 25-second mark where you will switch sides.

Make it easier: Use a lighter dumbbell.

Make it harder: Use a heavier dumbbell.

# Lunges with a Twist

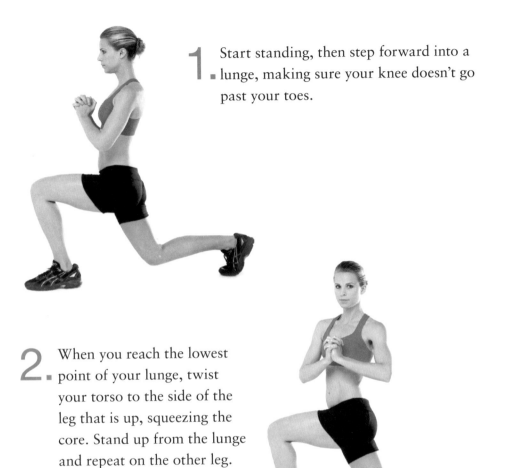

1. Start standing, then step forward into a lunge, making sure your knee doesn't go past your toes.

2. When you reach the lowest point of your lunge, twist your torso to the side of the leg that is up, squeezing the core. Stand up from the lunge and repeat on the other leg.

Make it easier: Don't sink as low in your lunge.

Make it harder: Lunge holding a dumbbell in front of your chest for extra difficulty.

# Sumo Squat with Dumbbell

**1.** Stand with feet about twice as wide as your shoulders, toes turned out slightly, holding a dumbbell ball in both hands at waist height.

**2.** Squat as low as you can, keeping a natural arch in the lower back, as if you are going to touch the weight to the ground between your feet.

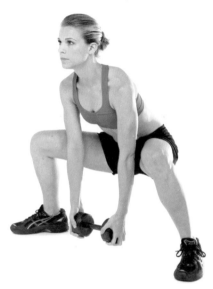

**3.** Come back up to the starting position and repeat. Keep the core engaged, focus the weight into your heels, and squeeze your glutes as you rise, pushing through the toes to work the calves as well.

Make it easier: Skip the weight.

Make it harder: As you come up to standing position, lift the weight over your head until your arms are straight, for 1 complete rep.

# Fire Hydrant

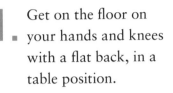

1. Get on the floor on your hands and knees with a flat back, in a table position.

2. Keeping your knee bent, lift one knee up and out to the side. Try to lift the knee as high as your hip, or whatever height is comfortable, squeezing the glutes.

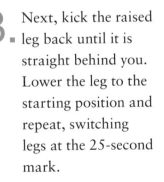

3. Next, kick the raised leg back until it is straight behind you. Lower the leg to the starting position and repeat, switching legs at the 25-second mark.

Make it easier: Skip the kick back.

Make it harder: Extend the opposite arm out in front of you.

# Side Leg Raise

**1.** Lie on your left side on the floor and rest your head in the crook of your elbow. Place your right hand in front of your body for stability.

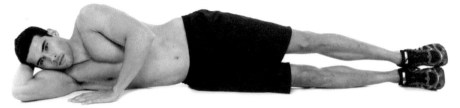

**2.** Keeping your body still, use the inner and outer thigh muscles and glutes to lift your right leg straight up as high as you can. Pause for a second at the top, then lower the leg to the starting position and repeat, switching legs at the 25-second mark.

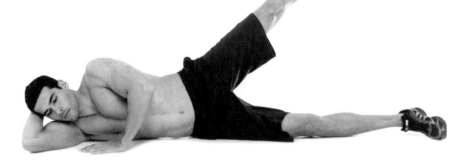

Make it easier: Don't lift the leg as high.

Make it harder: Perform 3 pulses at the top of the exercise, further engaging the inner thigh.

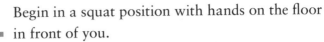

# Burpees

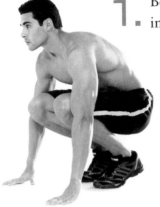

**1.** Begin in a squat position with hands on the floor in front of you.

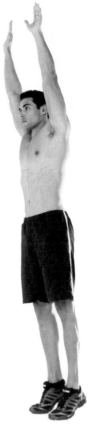

**2.** Kick your feet back into a push-up position without letting your hips sag. Immediately jump your feet back to the squat position.

**3.** Jump straight up as high as you can for 1 complete rep.

Make it easier: Walk your feet back into push-up position. Reach up instead of jumping up.

Make it harder: Kick your feet back, while simultaneously lowering yourself down into a push-up. Jump as high as you can each time.

# Bridge Pose and Curl On Stability Ball

1. Lie on your back on the floor with your feet and calves resting on a stability ball. Have your arms resting easily out to the sides.

2. Using your core and glutes, lift your hips off the ground so your body forms a straight line.

3. Curl the stability ball in toward your butt with your heels, as close as you can get it without arching your lower back. Your hips should stay in line with your body. Then, slide the ball back out and lower the hips to the ground for 1 rep.

Make it easier: Skip the curl and just raise the hips up and down.

Make it harder: Turn in the toes on the stability. ball to work the inner legs more.

# Cardio Plan

**Equipment:**
None

Combining strength training with cardiovascular exercise is the best way to lose weight quickly, safely, and easily. After performing the core, upper, or lower body exercises prescribed for the day, choose a cardio activity. The cardio portion of this plan includes one running and one walking interval for blasting calories in a short amount of time; choose from one of those custom programs, or pick your own cardio activity of 30 minutes or more.

Whatever you choose, from walking to hiking to kickboxing to surfing, be sure the activity is vigorous enough to get your heart rate up. When you reach your target heart rate, which is 60 to 70 percent of your maximum heart rate, you are in the zone when your body burns the most calories and body fat stores.

## Cardio Pyramid

This cardio workout will take 30 minutes. You will combine shorts bursts of jogging, running, and sprinting with periods of active recovery. You can adjust speeds as needed, but try to challenge yourself. Active recovery can be either a gentle jog or walk. Sprinting should be running almost as fast as you can. For an extra challenge, you can do this workout where there are uphill sections.

| TIME | ACTIVITY | RECOVER |
|---|---|---|
| 5 min. | walk or jog | 0 |
| 1 min. | run | 1 |
| 30 sec. | sprint | 30 sec. |
| 15 sec. | sprint | 15 sec. |
| 1 min. | run | 1 |
| 1 min. | sprint | 1 |
| 3.5 min. | jog or run | 3.5 |
| 1 min. | sprint | 1 |
| 1 min. | run | 1 |
| 15 sec. | sprint | 15 sec. |
| 30 sec. | sprint | 30 sec. |
| 1 min. | run | 1 |
| 5 min. | walk or jog | 0 |

## Walking Hills Workout

Walking is low-impact but still packs a calorie-burning punch, especially when walking at various speeds. A slow walk is for warming up and periods of active recovery. A moderate walk should get your heart rate up and have you moving briskly. A fast walk should mean you are working your hardest, raising your heart rate, and feeling a burn in the legs and glutes.

Be sure to pump your arms and keep your core tight and back straight. Here is a 30-minute walking workout you can do anywhere.

| MINUTES | ACTIVITY |
|:---:|:---:|
| 5 | warm-up |
| 2 | moderate walk |
| 2 | fast walk |
| 1 | slow walk |
| 1 | fast walk |
| 4 | moderate walk |
| 2 | slow walk |
| 2 | fast walk |
| 3 | moderate walk |
| 3 | fast walk |
| 5 | cool-down |

## Group Class, Activity, or Sport of Your Choice

You may also choose the physical activity you want to do as your cardio for the day. Be sure to challenge yourself and engage in an activity, class, or sport that lasts 30 to 60 minutes and gets your heart rate up, such as:

| MINUTES | ACTIVITY |
|:---:|:---:|
| 30-60 | Cardio kickboxing class |
| 30-60 | Swimming |
| 30-60 | Challenging hike |
| 30-60 | Vigorous bike ride |
| 30-60 | Surfing |
| 30-60 | Tennis |
| 30-60 | Yoga flow class |
| 30-60 | Aerobics class |
| 30-60 | Spinning |
| 30-60 | Running/climbing stairs |

# 16

"When the grass looks greener on
the other side of the fence, it may be
that they take better care of it there."
~ Unknown

# Lose Weight Fast Diet
# Meal Plan

**Never think of eating healthier as depriving** yourself of your favorite foods! The *Lose Weight Fast Diet* Meal Plan has been custom-created by our registered dietician and nutrition specialist, Lindsey Toth, to provide healthy, delicious meals, all low in saturated fats and containing about 400 calories each. Additionally, a list of snacks (all with 200 calories or less) rounds out your daily intake. Deciding what to eat is easy with this meal plan because you can mix and match from 20 breakfasts, 20 lunches, 20 dinners, and 20 snacks. Find your favorites, from smoothies to paninis to pizza.

Lindsey Toth, MS, RD is a nationally recognized registered dietitian and nutritionist for PepsiCo's Global Nutrition Communications Team. She graduated from Michigan State University's Honors College with degrees in dietetics and nutritional sciences, and holds a master's from Tufts University in clinical nutrition and nutrition communications. Her expertise has been tapped for *Redbook*, *Nutrition Today*, *The Dr. Oz Show*, and more.

# Apple Strudel Oatmeal

**Prep Time:** 7 minutes, **Total Time:** 10 minutes

Did your mom ever tell you no dessert for breakfast? Well we're flipping that rule on its head with this recipe. Warm, sweet, and ever so delicious, this oatmeal is the perfect start to your day.

### Ingredients:

- ½ cup dried, old-fashioned oats
- 1 cup fat-free milk
- ½ apple, cored, and diced
- ½ tsp cinnamon
- ½ tsp brown sugar
- 2 tbsps of crushed & roasted, unsalted pecans

### Nutrition Information:

Parfait:
371 calories
56 g carbohydrates
8 g fiber
15 g protein
11 g fat
1 g saturated fat

### Directions:

1. Portion dried oatmeal into a bowl and mix in milk, cinnamon, and brown sugar.

2. Stir in diced apple and microwave on high for 3 minutes, stirring occasionally.

3. Mix in crushed pecans and enjoy!

**Did You Know:**
There are more than 7,500 varieties of apples grown in the world, and about 2,500 varieties grown in the United States. Each variety has its own unique flavor (Fuji are sweet, Braeburn are tart, etc.), so test out different kinds in your oatmeal to find the taste that's right for you!

# PB&J Oatmeal

**Prep Time:** 0 minutes, **Total Time:** 3 minutes

Sweet, savory, and packed with protein, this PB&J has been mixed up oatmeal-style for a fun breakfast treat.

## Directions:

1. Portion dried oatmeal into a bowl and mix in milk, cinnamon, and scoop in peanut butter.

2. Microwave according to directions on oatmeal container (about 2-3 minutes).

3. Stir to mix in peanut butter, top with preserves, and mix well.

## Ingredients:

- ½ cup dried, old-fashioned oats
- 1 cup water
- 2 tbsps peanut butter
- ⅛ tsp cinnamon
- 2 tbsps Smucker's sugar free strawberry preserves

## Nutrition Information:

Parfait:
362 calories
46 g carbohydrates
6 g fiber
12 g protein
18 g fat
3 g saturated fat

**Did You Know:**

Peanut butter came into existence, because Dr. John Harvey Kellogg, a physician, wanted to help patients eat more plant-based protein, so he patented his procedure for making peanut butter in 1895.

# South of the Border Breakfast Sandwich

**Prep Time:** 7 minutes, **Total Time:** 10 minutes

This breakfast gem has all the magical zing of a breakfast burrito without the supersized portion and crazy calories. The salsa will put pep in your morning step and the protein-packed egg whites and lean turkey will keep you focused and satisfied until lunch.

## Ingredients:

- 1 whole wheat English muffin
- 2 oz 98% fat-free deli turkey (usually 3-4 slices or 56 grams)
- 3 egg whites (or the equivalent in carton egg substitutes)
- 1 tbsp of shredded, low-fat mozzarella cheese
- ¼ cup fresh baby spinach leaves (or ⅛ cup thawed frozen spinach)
- 1 tbsp salsa
- Olive oil cooking spray

## Nutrition Information:

Parfait: 371 calories, 56 g carbohydrates, 8 g fiber, 15 g protein, 11 g fat, 1 g saturated fat

## Directions:

1. Cut English muffin in half and place in toaster until toasted.

2. While muffin is toasting, pour egg whites in a small bowl, whisking in mozzarella with a fork. Add in spinach and stir completely.

3. Spray a coffee mug with cooking spray and pour egg mixture into mug.

4. Microwave egg mixture on high for 1:30 to 2 minutes, checking occasionally until done (eggs should form a slightly domed patty shape when done).

5. Remove egg cup from microwave and place egg patty on one side of toasted English muffin. Place turkey slices on other side and top with salsa. Put halves together and enjoy!

# Huevos Rancheros

Prep Time: 6 minutes, Total Time: 20 minutes

This is a classic Mexican breakfast dish, with a low calorie twist. Try this recipe on a weekend morning, or a morning when you have enough time to get your oven going.

## Directions

1. Preheat oven to 400°F.

2. Combine beans, lime juice, cumin, and olive oil in a small bowl.

3. Spray both sides of tortilla with olive oil cooking spray and bake in oven until crisp, about 10 minutes.

4. Spray frying pan lightly with olive oil cooking spray and add in eggs. Cook until whites are set, about 3 minutes.

5. Plate egg on top of tortilla, and top with beans, avocado, salsa, and cilantro.

## Ingredients

- 2 eggs
- 1 La Tortilla Factory 100% Whole Wheat 50 Calorie Tortilla
- ⅛ cup canned black beans, rinsed to remove excess sodium
- ½ tsp lime juice
- ¾ tsp olive oil
- ⅛ tsp ground cumin
- ¼ cup salsa
- ¼ of 1 avocado, peeled, pitted, and sliced
- Olive oil cooking spray
- 1 tsp cilantro

## Nutrition Information:

313 calories
25 g carbohydrates
9 g fiber
17 g protein
18 g fat
4 g saturated fat

# Zesty Pepper Packed Breakfast Roll-Up

**Prep Time:** 5 minutes, **Total Time:** 8 minutes

Packed with colorful peppers, this breakfast wrap is full of fiber, and vitamins A and B. It's also a snap to put together, and best of all, it's great if you're on the go!

## Ingredients:

- 1 La Tortilla Factory 100% Whole Wheat 100 Calorie Tortilla
- ¾ cup carton egg substitutes, like Egg Beaters (or 3 egg whites)
- 1 slice fat-free, white American cheese
- 1 cup frozen bell pepper, stir fry mix, reheated in microwave
- ¼ tsp red pepper
- 2 tbsps salsa
- Olive oil cooking spray

## Nutrition Information:

Total Meal: 258 calories

37 g carbohydrates

10 g fiber

29 g protein

2 g fat

0 g saturated fat

## Directions:

1. Spray a coffee mug or small bowl with cooking spray, and pour egg whites into mug.

2. Microwave eggs on high for 1:30 to 2 minutes, stirring occasionally until done to form a scramble.

3. Remove egg scramble from microwave and spread eggs onto one side of open tortilla, sprinkling with red pepper. Top with bell pepper mix, cheese, and salsa.

4. Roll into burrito form and microwave on high for another 15-20 seconds to melt cheese, and serve.

# Mean Green Breakfast Smoothie

**Prep Time:** 2 minutes, **Total Time:** 7 minutes

The color of this smoothie may be a bit off-putting, but the nutritional benefits aren't. This smoothie is chock-full of cancer-fighting phytochemicals and anthocyanins, satiating protein, and sweet delicious goodness. If you're in a jam to get out the door ASAP in the morning, this smoothie is a quick way to fit in the most important meal of the day.

## Directions:

1. Combine milk, yogurt, berries, sweet potato, and spinach in a blender.

2. Blend until smooth.

3. Pour into glass and enjoy.

## Ingredients:

- 1 cup fat-free milk
- 1 6-oz container of nonfat vanilla Greek yogurt
- ½ cup mixed, frozen berries
- ¼ raw sweet potato
- 1 cup chopped, frozen spinach

## Nutrition Information:
Parfait:
319 calories
49 g carbohydrates
7 g fiber
31 g protein
1 g fat
0 g saturated fat

## Did You Know:

Fresh spinach slowly loses its nutritional value after harvested. While fresh, its leaves are crisp and vibrant, but as it deteriorates, the leaves turn limp. Freeze spinach while fresh to preserve its high nutrient profile.

# Banana Split Smoothie

**Prep Time:** 2 minutes, **Total Time:** 7 minutes

This may seem reminiscent of a banana split, but the protein it's packing is definitely not: 17 grams to fill you up and keep you satisfied until lunch time. And chocolate for breakfast – what's not to love?

## Ingredients:

- 1 cup fat-free milk
- ½ cup mixed, frozen strawberries
- 1 banana
- 2 tbsps peanut butter
- 2 tbsps no sugar added Nesquik

## Nutrition Information:

375 calories
44 g carbohydrates
6 g fiber
17 g protein
17 g fat
4 g saturated fat

## Directions

1. Combine milk, berries, banana, peanut butter, and Nesquik powder in a blender.

2. Blend until smooth.

3. Pour into glass and enjoy.

**Did You Know:**

The browner the banana is, the sweeter it tastes? If some of your bananas are going brown, throw them in the freezer instead of the trash, and save them for smoothies. When you're ready to make your smoothie, remove the banana from the freezer, microwave it for 15-20 seconds, rip off the tip, and just squeeze the thawed banana into your blender.

# Fruit & Yogurt Roll-Up

**Prep Time:** 2 minutes, **Total Time:** 8 minutes

Not feeling like a savory, egg and cheese breakfast burrito? This fruit and yogurt burrito is the perfect solution: sweet, crunchy, and packed with protein, it practically screams "wake-up call."

## Directions

1. Spread cream cheese on tortilla. Top with Greek yogurt, oats, and nuts.

2. Microwave berries to thaw if still frozen and add to tortilla.

3. Roll tightly to prevent yogurt spillage, and enjoy.

## Ingredients:

- 1 La Tortilla Factory 100% Whole Wheat 100 Calorie Tortilla
- ½ ounce fat-free cream cheese
- 3 oz fat-free vanilla Greek yogurt
- 1 tbsp dried, old-fashioned oats
- 1 tbsp crushed walnuts
- 1 cup of frozen mixed berries, thawed

## Nutrition Information:

Parfait: 363 calories
57 g carbohydrates
17 g fiber
26 g protein
7 g fat
1 g saturated fat

**Did You Know:**

Greek yogurt can contain up to 4 times the amount of protein as regular yogurt, and can be easier on the stomach for those with lactose-intolerance, as it has less lactose. Stick with the non-fat variety for a rich and creamy yogurt that's sure to satisfy both your taste buds and your waistline.

# Avocado Breakfast Toast

**Prep Time:** 10 minutes, **Total Time:** 15 minutes

There are a zillion ways to eat an avocado: topped on a salad, mixed as guacamole, rolled into sushi – the list is endless! My all-time favorite way to eat avocado though, is in an avocado breakfast toast. Use your chopping skills and take this toast for a morning test drive!

## Ingredients:

- 2 slices of whole wheat bread, toasted
- 2 tbsps Dijon honey mustard
- ½ avocado, peeled and sliced
- ½ tomato, thinly sliced
- 1 tbsp of dried basil
- Salt and pepper to taste

## Nutrition Information:

2 slices of toast
351 calories
45 g carbohydrates
12 g fiber
11 g protein
16 g fat
2 g saturated fat

## Directions:

1. Spread 1 tablespoon of the Dijon honey mustard on each piece of toast.

2. Add the avocado and the tomato slices evenly to each slice of toast.

3. Sprinkle both slices with basil and the salt and pepper to taste.

4. Eat with caution – this can get messy but it's definitely worth it!!

**Did You Know:**

The avocado is actually a fruit. Avocados provide nearly 20 essential nutrients to our bodies, including fiber, potassium, folic acid, vitamin E, and B vitamins, and also help our bodies absorb fat-soluble nutrients like alpha- and beta-carotene.

# Cinnamon Pumpkin Swirl Yogurt Parfait

Prep Time: 0 minutes, Total Time: 3 minutes

Ever find yourself wishing for fall? For the colorful leaves, the crisp cool air, and the fantastic fall food? Well wish no more, this parfait brings the spirit of fall straight to your kitchen, with antioxidant rich spices like cinnamon and nutmeg, mixed with nutrient-packed pumpkin and yogurt, you'll feel like you tripped and fell straight into November.

## Directions:

1. Scoop yogurt into a small bowl.

2. Stir in cinnamon, honey, vanilla, and pumpkin.

3. Top with almonds and oats, sprinkle with nutmeg, and enjoy!

## Ingredients:

- 6 oz non-fat plain Greek yogurt (¾ cup)
- ¼ tsp ground cinnamon
- 1 ½ tsp honey
- ¼ tsp vanilla
- 1 tbsp canned raw pumpkin
- 1 tbsp old fashioned oats
- 1 tbsp sliced almonds
- Dash of nutmeg

## Nutrition Information:

Parfait
322 calories
35 g carbohydrates
5 g fiber
25 g protein
11 g fat
1 g saturated fat

### Did You Know:

Research has shown that cinnamon has the highest antioxidant level of any of the spices, and even higher than many foods. There are as many antioxidants in 1 teaspoon of cinnamon as there are in an entire cup of pomegranate juice and as many as there are in ½ cup of blueberries!

# Egg and Bell Pepper Breakfast Scramble

**Prep Time:** 0 minutes, **Total Time:** 10 minutes

This breakfast scramble is packed full of B vitamins and vitamin A, and is super low in saturated fat – making it an excellent heart-healthy breakfast choice.

## Ingredients

- 2 pieces of whole wheat toast
- ¾ cup substitutes eggs like Egg Beaters
- ½ cup frozen mixed pepper stir-fry blend, thawed
- 1 slice fat-free Kraft white American cheese
- ½ tsp low sodium soy sauce
- ½ tsp minced garlic
- ¼ tsp ground black pepper
- Olive oil cooking spray

## Directions

1. Heat fry pan to medium heat and spray lightly with cooking spray.

2. Pour in eggs and scramble with garlic, black pepper, and soy sauce until 85% cooked.

3. Add in pepper/stir-fry mix and scramble until eggs are thoroughly cooked.

4. Gather egg mixture into a small bowl and portion on top of pieces of toast. Serve and enjoy.

**Nutrition Information:**
304 calories
37 g carbohydrates
6 g fiber
32 g protein
2 g fat
1 g saturated fat

# Tomato Muffin Breakfast Pizza

**Prep Time:** 3 minutes, **Total Time:** 8 minutes

This savory breakfast recipe is good mix-up to traditional cereal, and is chock-full of fiber and flavor.

## Directions

1. Cut English muffin in half.

2. Spread with ricotta cheese, top with tomato halves, and sprinkle with salt and pepper to taste.

3. Toast in toaster or conventional oven for 4-5 minutes, or until crispy.

## Ingredients

- 1 whole wheat English muffin
- 6 cherry tomatoes, cut in half
- 4 tbsps fat-free ricotta cheese
- ½ tsp dried basil
- Salt and pepper to taste

## Nutrition Information:

199 calories
35 g carbohydrates
7 g fiber
13 g protein
1 g fat
0 g saturated fat

**Did You Know:**

Do you know why breakfast is the most important meal of the day? The word breakfast literally means "breaking the fast of the night," as it's the first meal taken after a night's rest. This meal is needed to restock our body's energy stores, which have been depleted during the night, so we have energy for the day ahead.

# Maple-Almond Oatmeal

**Prep Time:** 0 minutes, **Total Time:** 5 minutes

This breakfast dish will transport you to the hills of Vermont with its tinge of maple-sweetness. The crunch of almonds will be sure to wake you up in the morning.

## Ingredients

- ½ cup dried, old-fashioned oats
- 1 cup water
- 1 tbsp sliced almonds
- 2 tbsps dried cranberries
- 1 tbsp maple syrup

## Nutrition Information:

325 calories
66 g carbohydrates
6 g fiber
7 g protein
6 g fat
1 g saturated fat

## Directions

1. Portion dried oatmeal into a bowl and mix in water.

2. Microwave on high for 3 minutes, stirring occasionally.

3. Mix in sliced almonds, dried cranberries, and maple syrup.

**Did You Know:**

Oatmeal is a good source of high-quality plant-based protein, zinc, copper, iron, managanese, vitamin E, and selenium, and is most famous for its high fiber content. The soluble fiber found in oatmeal has been found to lower LDL cholesterol (the bad cholesterol), and to help to stabilize blood sugar levels.

# Cereal Sundae

**Prep Time:** 0 minutes, **Total Time:** 3 minutes

A sundae for breakfast? In this case, absolutely! This breakfast sundae is full of fiber, calcium, and protein, perfect for your early morning wake-up call. Best of all, it's totally portable – mix your ingredients in a plastic container, snap on the lid, and head out to take on the day!

## Directions

1. Scoop yogurt into a small bowl.

2. Stir in bran cereal, almonds, and cranberries.

3. Serve and enjoy.

## Ingredients

- 6 oz non-fat vanilla Greek yogurt (3/4 cup)
- ½ cup bran flake cereal, like Raisin Bran
- 1 tbsp sliced almonds
- 1 tbsp dried cranberries

## Nutrition Information:

Parfait: 310 calories
43 g carbohydrates
5 g fiber
21 g protein
8 g fat
1 g saturated fat

## Did You Know:

Almonds are one of the best food sources of Vitamin E, and are a high source of calcium, magnesium, potassium, and a natural source of protein and fiber. A 1 ounce serving has 13 grams of good unsaturated fats, helping you maintain heart health.

# Fresh Berry Crêpes

**Prep Time:** 5 minutes, **Total Time:** 12 minutes

Think you have to head to France for crêpes? Think again! This breakfast meal is a fun and exotic way to incorporate fruit into your morning routine, and is a good source of B vitamins and fiber.

## Ingredients

- ¼ cup whole wheat flour
- 1 egg white (or ¼ cup egg substitute, like Egg Beaters)
- ¼ cup fat-free milk
- 1 ½ tsp cinnamon applesauce
- Dash of salt
- ½ tsp vanilla extract
- ½ cup mixed frozen berries, thawed
- Pinch of powdered sugar
- Cooking spray

## Nutrition Information:

Parfait: 204 calories
37 g carbohydrates
8 g fiber
13 g protein
1 g fat
0 g saturated fat

## Directions

1. In a small bowl, whisk together flour, egg, milk, applesauce, salt, and vanilla until smooth.

2. Heat frying pan on medium heat. Spray lightly with cooking spray to coat when heated.

3. Pour ½ of batter into skillet.

4. Tilt pan in circular motion to spread batter to edges, and cook until bottom is light brown, about 2 minutes.

5. Flip crêpe and fill with thawed mixed berries. Cook for another 2 minutes.

6. Fold crêpe in half and transfer to a plate.

7. Repeat with other half of batter for a second crêpe.

8. Dust crêpes lightly with powdered sugar and serve.

# Corn and Cheese Frittata

**Prep Time:** 10 minutes, **Total Time:** 18 minutes

This frittata is a delicious mixture of eggs and veggies, low in saturated fat, and high in B vitamins and vitamin A. Add in 34 grams of filling protein, and you're set to rock that morning meeting.

## Directions

1. Heat broiler-proof skillet over medium heat. Stir in olive oil, corn, zucchini, green onions, and tomatoes. Sauté for 3-5 minutes until vegetables are tender.

2. In a small bowl, mix together eggs and basil.

3. Pour egg mixture over vegetables in pan. As mixture sets, lift cooked portions so uncooked eggs flow underneath. Continue cooking until almost set. Sprinkle with cheese.

4. Place skillet in oven under broiler for 1-2 minutes or until top is set and cheese is melted.

## Ingredients

- 1 cup egg substitutes, like Egg Beaters
- 1 tsp olive oil
- ⅓ cup whole corn kernels
- ⅓ cup chopped zucchini
- ⅛ cup sliced green onions
- ⅓ cup diced tomatoes
- ⅛ cup fat-free cheddar cheese
- Olive oil cooking spray

## Nutrition Information:

284 calories
27 g carbohydrates
4 g fiber
34 g protein
6 g fat
1 g saturated fat

# Cranberry-Peanut Butter English Muffin

**Prep Time:** 0 minutes, **Total Time:** 6 minutes

Cut the traditional butter out of your muffin routine and replace it with protein-packed peanut butter. The whole wheat muffin delivers a healthy dose of fiber, the peanut butter provides hunger-relieving protein, and the cranberries top it off with a deliciously sweet tang.

## Ingredients

- 1 whole wheat English muffin
- 2 tbsps unsalted peanut butter
- 2 tbsps dried cranberries

## Nutrition Information:

370 calories
47 g carbohydrates
7 g fiber
13 g protein
17 g fat
3 g saturated fat

## Directions

1. Cut English muffin in half and spread each side with 1 tbsp of peanut butter.

2. Top each half with 1 tbsp of dried cranberries.

3. Toast in toaster or traditional oven until crispy, and serve.

**Did You Know:**

Looking to break away from your traditional peanut butter? Try mixing it up this morning with a different kind of nut butter, like almond or walnut butter. Both nut butters are as high in protein as peanut butter, and lower in saturated fat.

# Tropical Sunrise Oatmeal

**Prep Time:** 3 minutes, **Total Time:** 6 minutes

Is the cold weather giving you the vacation blues? Or maybe you just want to celebrate the fact that it's summer with an equally festive breakfast. Either way, this breakfast bowl is the perfect solution.

## Directions

1. Portion dried oatmeal into a bowl and mix in milk, vanilla extract, and pineapple.

2. Microwave on high for 3 minutes, stirring occasionally.

3. Mix in shredded coconut and enjoy!

## Ingredients

- ½ cup dried, old-fashioned oats
- 1 cup fat-free milk
- ½ cup canned pineapple, drained
- ¼ tsp vanilla extract
- 2 tbsp dried, sweetened, shredded coconut

## Nutrition Information:

Parfait: 337 calories
56 g carbohydrates
6 g fiber
14 g protein
7 g fat
4 g saturated fat

### Did You Know:

Some canned fruit, like canned pineapple, comes packed in syrup. This can significantly increase the calories you're consuming. When buying canned fruit, look for fruit that is canned in 100% juice for extra calorie savings. Want a flavor spin? Try using canned peaches, pears, or mandarin oranges instead of pineapple.

# Honey-Almond Fruit Salad

**Prep Time:** 15 minutes, **Total Time:** 20 minutes

This sweet and crunchy fruit salad is rich in antioxidants and fiber, and is a delicious start to any day.

## Ingredients

- ¼ medium banana, sliced
- ¼ cup fresh blueberries
- ¼ sliced strawberries
- ¼ cup fresh raspberries
- 2 tbsps sliced almonds
- ¼ tsp lemon juice
- ¼ tsp poppy seeds
- 1 ½ tsps honey

## Nutrition Information:

263 calories
31 g carbohydrates
7 g fiber
7 g protein
15 g fat
1 g saturated fat

## Directions

1. Combine banana, blueberries, strawberries, and raspberries in a small dish.

2. Mix together honey, lemon juice, poppy seeds, and almonds in a separate small bowl.

3. Pour lemon-honey mixture over fruit, and toss to coat.

**Did You Know:**

Try substituting 1 packet of no-calorie sweetener for the honey in this recipe. You'll knock the calories back an extra 32 calories, for an even lower calorie breakfast with the same great flavor. Some great no-calorie sweetener options include, Stevia, Splenda, and Equal, among others.

# Berry Crunchy Smoothie

**Prep Time:** 2 minutes, **Total Time:** 5 minutes

This breakfast smoothie is a great source of B vitamins. And the crunch along with the sweet, cold raspberries is sure to get your morning engine running.

## Directions

1. Combine milk, berries, banana, granola, and yogurt in a blender.

2. Blend until smooth (besides the occasional granola bit).

3. Pour into glass and enjoy.

## Ingredients

- 1 cup fat-free milk
- ½ cup mixed, frozen berries
- ½ medium banana
- ½ cup low-fat granola
- 3 oz vanilla non-fat Greek yogurt

## Nutrition Information:

397 calories
77 g carbohydrates
9 g fiber
19 g protein
3 g fat
1 g saturated fat

**Did You Know:**

Love mixed berries year round, but hate the cost spike during the winter months? If fresh berries are out of season in your area, remember that frozen berries provide the same nutritional punch as the fresh variety. Not only are frozen berries on par nutritionally with the fresh kind, but they often come at a lower cost as well.

# Fresh Peach & Chicken Spinach Salad

**Prep Time:** 10 minutes, **Total Time:** 15 minutes

This salad is a great lunch-time meal for those hot summer days, or even those cold winter ones when you're just wishing for the warmth of summer. Not only is it tasty, but this dish is also rich in vitamins A, C, and K, and low in calories to help you reach those weight-loss goals.

## Ingredients:

- 3 oz cooked, cubed chicken breast (about ½ cup)
- 1 small peach, pitted and cubed
- ¼ of one medium cucumber, cubed
- 1 cup fresh baby spinach leaves

### Vinaigrette:

- 1 tbsp white wine vinegar
- ¾ tsp lemon juice
- 1 tbsp sugar
- 1 tbsp fresh mint
- ⅛ tsp salt
- ⅛ tsp pepper

## Nutrition Information:

368 calories, 45 g carbohydrates, 5 g fiber, 16 g protein, 15 g fat, 3 g saturated fat

## Directions

1. Plate spinach leaves and top with peach cubes, chicken, and cucumber.

2. In a small bowl or dressing container, thoroughly mix together vinegar, lemon juice, sugar, mint, and salt.

3. Top chicken salad mixture with dressing, toss to coat, and serve.

# Crunchy PB&J Wrap

**Prep Time:** 8 minutes, **Total Time:** 8 minutes

Think peanut butter & jelly sandwiches are just for kids? Think again! Peanut butter is rich in protein, helping to keep you full until dinner. The fruit in this twist on a kid's classic is packed with disease-fighting antioxidants. So let your inner child out to play with this fun wrap!

## Directions

1. Spread tortilla with peanut butter and jelly.

2. Top with granola and mixed berries.

3. Roll and serve.

## Ingredients:

- 1 La Tortilla Factory 100% Whole Wheat 100 Calorie Tortilla
- 2 tbsps crunchy peanut butter, low or no added salt
- 2 tbsps sugar-free jelly or jam
- ⅛ cup low-fat granola
- ¼ cup mixed berries

## Nutrition Information:

403 calories
60 g carbohydrates
14 g fiber
14 g protein
18 g fat
3 g saturated fat

## Did You Know:

You don't have to chase after expensive international "superfoods" to get antioxidants in your diet – just head to your local produce aisle. For instance, did you know that broccoli contains many of the same anti-cancer properties as wheatgrass, but 25 times the vitamin C? Or that blueberry juice has an antioxidant capacity ranked higher than that of açaí berry juice?

# Toasted Chipotle Tuna Sandwich

**Prep Time:** 5 minutes, **Total Time:** 11 minutes

Subbing Greek yogurt for mayo in your tuna sandwich not only cuts back on fat and calories, but also ups the flavor factor and protein power. Throw in some chipotle chile pepper seasoning combined with a quick toasting to really heat things up.

## Ingredients:

- 1 sandwich thin
- 1 leaf of romaine lettuce
- 1-2 tomato slices
- 1 can of chunk light albacore tuna, in water
- ½ stick of celery, diced
- 1 tbsp of non-fat plain Greek yogurt
- ¼ tsp of ground black pepper
- ⅛ tsp lemon juice
- 2 ½ tsps honey Dijon mustard
- ¼ tsp chipotle chile pepper seasoning

## Nutrition Information:

334 calories
26 g carbohydrates
6 g fiber
49 g protein
2 g fat
0 g saturated fat

## Directions

1. Place lettuce and tomato on sandwich thin.

2. In a small bowl, mix rest of ingredients together.

3. Top sandwich with tuna mixture, close, and place in toaster oven until bread is toasted.

**Did You Know:**
The United States uses over 31% of the total amount of tuna caught in the world. Most of the tuna we consume is canned, which can come packed in either water, or oil. Both types can fit into a healthy diet, though tuna packed in water is slightly lower in calories (109 calories versus 158, for a 3-oz serving).

# Spinach Flatbread Pizza

**Prep Time:** 0 minutes, **Total Time:** 10 minutes

Let this flatbread pizza take you away from your kitchen and back to rustic Italy – sans the calories but rich in flavor.

## Directions

1. Preheat oven to 425°F.

2. Spray baking sheet lightly with cooking spray.

3. Place tortilla on baking sheet and spread with tomato sauce, leaving a small ring on outer edges as a crust.

4. Top with spinach, mushrooms, and mozzarella.

5. Bake pizza for 10 minutes, or until crust turns golden brown.

## Ingredients:

- 1 La Tortilla Factory 100% Whole Wheat 100 Calorie Tortilla
- ¼ cup tomato sauce
- ½ cup shredded, low-fat mozzarella cheese
- ½ cup frozen spinach, thawed and drained
- ½ cup chopped, white mushrooms

## Nutrition Information:

315 calories
37 g carbohydrates
12 g fiber
24 g protein
14 g fat
6 g saturated fat

### Did You Know:

You can now buy mushrooms fortified with Vitamin D! Three-quarters of U.S. teens and adults are deficient in Vitamin D, which is usually only found in animal foods, or received from sun exposure.

# Mediterranean Turkey Wrap

**Prep Time:** 2 minutes, **Total Time:** 10 minutes

Try this Mediterranean turkey wrap for a zesty, mid-day pick me up.

## Ingredients:

- 1 La Tortilla Factory 100% Whole Wheat 100 Calorie Tortilla
- 2 tbsps roasted red pepper hummus
- 2 oz 98% fat free deli turkey (usually 3-4 slices or 56 grams)
- ½ cup alfalfa sprouts
- ½ cup fresh baby spinach
- ⅛ cup Athenos Reduced Fat Feta Cheese
- 2 fresh basil leaves, shredded
- 4 cherry tomatoes, sliced in half

## Nutrition Information:

282 calories
34 g carbohydrates
12 g fiber
23 g protein
8 g fat
1 g saturated fat

## Directions

1. Spread hummus in middle of tortilla wrap and place turkey on top.

2. Cover with sprouts, spinach, feta, basil, and cherry tomatoes.

3. Roll up tortilla and enjoy.

**Did You Know:**
The health benefits of a Mediterranean-based diet are well known, with hummus among one of the top contributors. Hummus contains chickpeas, which are a great source of soluble fiber, and help to lower cholesterol. Want more ways to incorporate hummus into your diet? Try substituting it for mayonnaise in sandwiches, for cream cheese on bagels, or as a dip with fresh vegetables.

# Sweet Potato Panini with Strawberry Spinach Salad

**Prep Time:** 3 minutes, **Total Time:** 11 minutes

Don't let the sweet potato fool you, this sandwich has a real kick to it thanks to the red pepper hummus. The salad is just the right amount of sweet and savory to tickle your taste buds.

## Directions

1. Heat frying pan on medium heat.

2. While pan is heating, spread sandwich thins with hummus (1 tbsp on each side) and top with 7-8 spinach leaves, sprouts, and avocado.

3. Spray heated pan lightly with cooking spray, and place the 4 sweet potato slices in pan. Spray tops of slices lightly with cooking spray. Grill for 3 minutes on each side, or until soft.

4. While sweet potato slices are cooking, plate 1 cup of spinach and top with strawberries, walnuts, and light vinaigrette (try Newman's Own Organic Light Balsamic Dressing at only 23 calories per tbsp).

5. Remove sweet potato from pan, sprinkle lightly with sea salt and pepper, and place on sandwich. Serve toasted if preferred.

## Ingredients:

**Sandwich:**
- ¼ of a large sweet potato cut into 4 ¼ inch discs
- 2 tbsps of red pepper hummus
- 1 sandwich thin
- ½ cup alfalfa sprouts
- 7-8 baby spinach leaves
- Salt and pepper

**Salad:**
- 1 cup of baby spinach
- 3 strawberries, sliced
- 1 tsp crushed walnuts
- 1 tbsp light balsamic vinaigrette

## Nutrition Information:

**Salad:** 92 calories, 6 g carbohydrates, 2 g fiber, 2 g protein, 7 g fat, 1 g saturated fat

**Sandwich:** 274 calories, 38 g carbohydrates, 12 g fiber, 10 g protein, 12 g fat, 1 g saturated fat

**Total Meal:** 366 calories, 44 g carbohydrates, 15 g fiber, 12 g protein, 19 g fat, 2 g saturated fat

# Crispy Club Sandwich

**Prep Time:** 6 minutes, **Total Time:** 11 minutes

Thoughts of restaurant club sandwiches may send shivers up and down your spine (calories and fat – oh my!). But this version is low in both, and is also a good source of vitamin C – who would've thought?! Pack this for lunch the night before and reheat it at lunch for a meal with restaurant style flavor with made-at-home calories.

## Ingredients

- 2 slices of whole wheat bread, toasted
- 2 slices of Jennie-O Extra Lean Turkey Bacon, cooked
- 2 oz 98% fat-free deli turkey
- 2 slices of tomato
- 2 leaves of romaine lettuce
- 2 tsps fat-free mayonnaise

## Nutrition Information:

279 calories
32 g carbohydrates
6 g fiber
26 g protein
5 g fat
1 g saturated fat

## Directions

1. Spread each slice of bread with 1 tsp of mayonnaise.

2. Top one slice with turkey, bacon, tomato, and lettuce.

3. Close sandwich and serve.

**Did You Know:**

The average club sandwich can run up to 700 calories and 30-40 grams of fat?! Be wary of sandwiches packed with mayo, as their calories and fat can be off the charts and way out of your calorie budget for the day. This sandwich swap is a good alternative to the traditional restaurant club.

# Southwest-Style Chicken Sandwich

**Prep Time:** 8 minutes, **Total Time:** 15 minutes

This sandwich adds a fun, Southwestern flavor to your day, while packing in the protein, B vitamins and vitamin C.

## Directions

1. Mix together ingredients for Southwest sauce in a small bowl.

2. Spread slices of bread with Southwest sauce.

3. Mix together chicken, tomatoes, green pepper, and onion in a bowl, and top mixture on one slice of bread.

4. Place slice of cheese on top of chicken mixture.

5. Close sandwich and toast in toaster or conventional oven for 3-4 minutes, or until toasted and the cheese is melted.

## Ingredients

**Sandwich:**
- 2 slices of whole wheat bread
- 3 oz cooked chicken breast, diced
- ⅛ cup diced tomatoes
- ⅛ cup diced green pepper
- ⅛ cup diced onion
- 1 slice fat-free shredded white American cheese

**Southwest** Sauce:
- ⅛ cup fat-free mayonnaise
- ¼ tsp spicy Dijon mustard
- ¼ tsp lime juice
- ⅛ tsp chipotle chile pepper
- ⅛ tsp minced garlic

## Nutrition Information:
306 calories, 35 g carbohydrates, 5 g fiber, 32 g protein, 4 g fat, 1 g saturated fat

# Tarragon Potato Chicken Salad

**Prep Time:** 15 minutes, **Total Time:** 20 minutes

This chicken salad is low in saturated fat, but packed with protein, vitamins, minerals, and flavor. Go ahead and serve it cold or warm – it's delicious either way!

Ingredients
- 4 oz cooked, cubed chicken breast (about ½ cup)
- 1 cup baby spinach leaves
- ½ cup chopped snap peas
- 1 small, red skin potato, chopped
- ¼ cup chopped red bell pepper
- 2 tbsps chopped red onion
- ½ tbsp olive oil
- ½ tbsp white wine vinegar
- ¾ tsp lemon juice
- ¾ tsp Dijon mustard
- ¼ tsp dried tarragon
- ¼ tsp salt
- ⅛ tsp ground black pepper
- ¼ tsp minced garlic

**Nutrition Information:**
361 calories, 38 g carbohydrates, 6 g fiber, 32 g protein, 9 g fat, 1 g saturated fat

Directions
1. Place potato and snap peas in a microwave safe bowl, pour in 1 tbsp of water, cover partially, and microwave on high for 4-5 minutes, or until tender.

2. Place spinach leaves, potato, and snap peas in a small salad bowl. Top with chicken, bell pepper, and onion.

3. In a small bowl or dressing container, thoroughly mix together olive oil, white wine vinegar, lemon juice, mustard, tarragon, salt, pepper, and garlic.

4. Top chicken salad with dressing, toss to coat, and serve.

# Chicken Waldorf Salad

**Prep Time:** 15 minutes, **Total Time:** 20 minutes

This salad is everything you could ask for in a lunch: sweet, crunchy, low in calories, and bursting at the seams with flavor. Top it off with 22 grams of satiating protein and you've got yourself a brown-bag winner!

## Directions

1. Toss apple slices with lemon juice.

2. Toss remaining ingredients with apple slices in a salad bowl.

3. Drizzle raspberry vinaigrette over salad. Serve and enjoy.

## Ingredients

- 3 oz chicken breast, boneless, skinless, diced (cooked)
- 2 cups mixed salad greens
- ¼ tsp lemon juice
- ½ cup chopped Gala apples
- ¼ cup green grapes, halved
- 2 tbsps chopped celery
- 2 tbsps chopped walnuts
- 2 tbsps dried cherries
- ¼ of 1 red onion, thinly sliced
- 2 tbsps reduced-fat raspberry vinaigrette

## Nutrition Information:

305 calories, 37 g carbohydrates, 4 g fiber, 22 g protein, 8 g fat, 1 g saturated fat

**Did You Know:**

Tart cherries, whether enjoyed dried or frozen, have among the highest levels of disease-fighting antioxidants, when compared with other fruits. They also contain other important nutrients like beta-carotene (19 times more than blueberries or strawberries), vitamin C, magnesium, potassium, iron, folate, and fiber.

# Avocado Bean Sandwich

**Prep Time:** 8 minutes, **Total Time:** 10 minutes

**A** great option for vegetarians, this sandwich is flavorful and full of heart-healthy fats and fiber.

## Ingredients

- 1 Arnold Select 100% Whole Wheat Sandwich Thin
- ½ cup canned white beans, rinsed to remove excess sodium
- ½ tsp olive oil
- ⅛ tsp salt
- ⅛ tsp ground black pepper
- 3 thin slices of red onion
- 4 cucumber slices, with peel
- ½ cup alfalfa sprouts
- ½ avocado, pitted and sliced

## Nutrition Information:

387 calories
55 g carbohydrates
17 g fiber
17 g protein
14 g fat
2 g saturated fat

## Directions

1. In a small bowl, mash together beans, olive oil, salt, and pepper. Spread mixture onto sandwich thin.

2. Top with red onion, cucumber, alfalfa sprouts, and avocado.

3. Close sandwich and serve.

# Halibut Salad

**Prep Time:** 15 minutes, **Total Time:** 20 minutes

This salad is a refreshingly low-calorie lunch-time treat, and is a great way to incorporate more fish into your diet. Try this with a number of different fish fillets (salmon, tuna, tilapia, etc.) to find the flavor that really works for you.

## Directions

1. Season fish with salt and pepper to taste, and simmer in ½ inch of water on medium-high heat to cook, about 6-8 minutes.

2. Set fish aside to cool, and flake into large pieces.

3. Plate salad greens and top with halibut pieces, chickpeas, avocado, and red onion.

4. In a small bowl or dressing container, thoroughly mix together olive oil, lemon juice, mustard, cilantro, salt, and pepper.

5. Drizzle salad with vinaigrette and serve.

## Ingredients

Salad:
- 1 3 oz piece of halibut
- Salt and pepper to taste
- 2 cups mixed salad greens
- ¼ cup canned chickpeas, rinsed to remove excess sodium
- ¼ avocado, peeled and pitted
- 3 slices of red onion

Vinaigrette:
- 1 tbsp olive oil
- ½ tsp lemon juice
- ½ tsp Dijon mustard
- ½ tbsp fresh chopped cilantro
- ⅛ tsp salt
- ⅛ ground black pepper

## Nutrition Information:

292 calories, 21 g carbohydrates, 7 g fiber, 24 g protein, 13 g fat, 2 g saturated fat

# Chilled Shrimp Salad

**Prep Time:** 15 minutes, **Total Time:** 20 minutes

This shrimp salad is a delicious and simple addition to your meal plan for the day. Topped with flavor-bursting feta cheese and cilantro, it's sure to lighten up your plate – and your calorie load for the day.

## Ingredients

- 2 cups mixed salad greens
- 3.5 oz cooked and peeled shrimp
- ¼ cup chopped cucumber
- ¼ cup diced tomato
- ¼ cup canned chickpeas, rinsed to remove excess sodium
- 2 tbsps Athenos Reduced Fat Feta Cheese
- 2 tsps olive oil
- ½ tsp cilantro
- ½ tbsp red wine vinegar
- Dash of salt and pepper to taste

## Nutrition Information:

387 calories, 17 g carbohydrates, 6 g fiber, 39 g protein, 16 g fat, 4 g saturated fat

## Directions

1. Toss all ingredients together in a small bowl. Serve chilled.

**Did You Know:**

4 ounces of shrimp provides almost half the daily requirement of vitamin D, also known as the "sunshine vitamin." Vitamin D helps us build strong bones, maintain a healthy immune system, and may also lower the risk of certain conditions like type 2 diabetes and high blood pressure.

# Greek Salad Pita

Prep Time: 6 minutes, Total Time: 8 minutes

This pita is the perfect way to enjoy your Greek salad on the go, and it's packed full of fiber to help you stay full until dinner time.

## Directions

1. In a small bowl, mix together lettuce, feta cheese, cherry tomatoes, red onion lemon juice, and parmesan cheese.

2. Cut an opening in pita, fill with salad mixture, and serve.

**Did You Know:**

The term "Greek salad" is used in North America to refer to a salad with Greek-inspired ingredients, dressed with oil and vinegar. The most standard elements are lettuce, tomatoes, feta cheese, and olives, with additional ingredients that vary on location. In Detroit, Michigan, for example, a "Greek salad" also includes beets, and in Tampa Bay, Florida, it often includes potato salad.

## Ingredients

- 1 Joseph's Flax, Oat Bran & Whole Wheat Pita
- 1 ½ cups shredded romaine lettuce
- ⅛ cup Athenos Reduced Fat Feta Cheese
- 6 cherry tomatoes, sliced in half
- ⅛ cup chopped red onion
- 1 tbsp fat-free parmesan cheese
- 1 tbsp lemon juice

## Nutrition Information:

293 calories
29 g carbohydrates
8 g fiber
26 g protein
8 g fat
3 g saturated fat

# Mandarin Mango Chicken Salad

**Prep Time:** 15 minutes, **Total Time:** 20 minutes

The sweet tang of mandarin oranges combined with the fantastic crunch of broccoli makes this salad the perfect mid-afternoon wake-up call for lunch.

## Ingredients

**Salad:**

- 3 oz chicken breast, boneless, skinless, cooked and diced
- 1 cup chopped broccoli florets, raw
- ¼ of one large mango, diced
- 2 tbsps cashews, salt-free, chopped
- ¼ of 1 red onion, thinly sliced

**Dressing:**

- 2 tbsps Ranch dressing, reduced fat
- ½ tbsp orange juice
- ¼ tbsp horseradish

## Nutrition Information:

337 calories
27 g carbohydrates
2 g fiber
22 g protein
17 g fat
3 g saturated fat

## Directions

1. Grill raw chicken breast in frying pan until done, about 5 minutes.

2. Toss remaining salad ingredients and grilled chicken in a salad bowl.

3. In a small container with a lid, mix together dressing ingredients thoroughly.

4. Drizzle salad dressing over salad. Serve and enjoy.

**Did You Know:**

Mango is delicious but can be a challenge to cut. Try these steps: 1) Cut ends off of mango, and stand on end. 2) Cut down each side to remove meat, avoiding the pit in the middle. 3) Make lengthwise and crosswise cuts in mango sides, avoiding the peel. 4) Peel mango segments off peel.

# Salad Niçoise

**Prep Time:** 15 minutes, **Total Time:** 30 minutes

Niçoise salad is a traditional French salad named for the city of Nice. It consists of vegetables, flaked tuna or salmon, and anchovies.

## Directions

1. Toss all salad ingredients together in a small bowl.

2. In a small container with a lid, mix dressing ingredients thoroughly.

3. Drizzle salad dressing over salad. Serve and enjoy.

### Did You Know:

The American Heart Association recommends eating salmon or other fatty fish twice a week for the heart-protective benefits associated with the omega-3 fatty acids found in fish oils. There are nutritional differences between farm-raised and wild-caught, as farmed salmon generally contains more calories, more fat, and more omega-3 fatty acids than wild salmon.

## Ingredients

**Salad:**
- 2 cups mixed salad greens
- ¼ cup fresh green beans
- ¼ cup flaked cooked salmon (fresh or canned)
- ½ medium tomato, cut into wedges
- 1 hardboiled egg, sliced
- 1 tbsp diced green onions
- 1 anchovy fillet, rinsed, and patted dry

**Dressing:**
- 1 tbsp olive oil
- 1 tbsp white wine vinegar
- ¼ tsp honey
- ¼ tsp Dijon mustard
- Dash of salt and pepper
- ⅛ tsp dried tarragon

**Nutrition Information:**
325 calories, 9 g carbohydrates, 5 g fiber, 18 g protein, 24 g fat, 5 g saturated fat

# Tarragon Lime Chicken and Bacon Wrap

**Prep Time:** 8 minutes, **Total Time:** 12 minutes

This zesty chicken wrap is a great source of fiber and protein, and is packed with vitamins A, B6, and K. It's also low in saturated fat, making it a great heart-healthy and low-calorie lunch choice.

## Ingredients

- 1 La Tortilla Factory 100% Whole Wheat 100 Calorie Tortilla
- 2 tbsps fat-free mayonnaise
- ½ tsp lemon juice
- ¼ tsp dried tarragon
- ½ cup shredded lettuce
- ½ cup chopped tomato
- 1 slice of Jennie-O's Extra Lean Turkey Bacon, cooked
- 4 oz diced chicken breast, skinless boneless, cooked (about ½ cup)

## Nutrition Information:

284 calories
32 g carbohydrates
10 g fiber
35 g protein
4 g fat
1 g saturated fat

## Directions

1. In a small dish, mix together mayonnaise, tarragon, and lemon juice.

2. Spread mayo mixture down the middle of tortilla wrap and top with chicken, lettuce, and tomato. Crumble bacon on top.

3. Roll up tortilla and enjoy.

**Did You Know:**

The name "tarragon" comes from the French word estragon, which means "little dragon." Some think the herb was given this name for its supposed ability to cure venomous reptile bites. Tarragon has a pleasant licorice-like aroma, with a bittersweet taste, and is great paired with chicken, fish, egg, or vegetable dishes.

# Chicken Shawarma

**Prep Time:** 20 minutes, **Total Time:** 40 minutes

This middle-eastern dish is a delicious, flavor-packed lunch to prepare the night before, and reheat at noon the next day.

## Directions

1. Heat frying pan on medium heat.

2. While pan heats up, stir together lemon juice, curry powder, olive oil, salt cumin, and garlic.

3. Toss chicken in mixture to coat. Refrigerate for 20 minutes to let marinate.

4. Prepare sauce by mixing together yogurt, tahini, lemon juice, garlic, and dash of salt.

5. Remove chicken from refrigerator, spray frying pan lightly with olive oil cooking spray, and place in frying pan. Cook chicken until done, turning occasionally. Remove chicken from pan when done.

6. Re-spray frying pan with cooking oil. Place pitas in pan and grill each side lightly, about 1 minute per side.

7. Place grilled pita on plate, top with grilled chicken, lettuce, tomato, and sauce.

## Ingredients

- 1 Joseph's Flax, Oat Bran & Whole Wheat Pita
- ¼ cup shredded romaine lettuce
- 2 tomato slices
- Olive oil cooking spray
- 4 oz chicken breast, skinless, boneless, cut into strips
- ½ tbsp lemon juice
- ¼ tsp curry powder
- ½ tsp olive oil
- ⅛ tsp salt
- ⅛ tsp ground cumin
- ¾ tsp of minced garlic

**Sauce:**
- 2 tbsps non-fat, plain Greek yogurt
- ½ tbsp tahini
- ½ tsp lemon juice
- ¼ tsp of minced garlic
- Dash of salt

## Nutrition Information:
282 calories, 15 g carbohydrates, 5 g fiber, 37 g protein, 10 g fat, 1 g saturated fat

# Turkey Bacon Melt

**Prep Time:** 7 minutes, **Total Time:** 12 minutes

The name of this recipe may make you think of fat, fat, and more fat, but this low-cal spin will change your mind. This melt is actually low in saturated fat, but still packed with the cheesy, gooey flavor you've come to love in a sandwich melt.

## Ingredients

- 2 slices of whole wheat bread
- 2 slices of Jennie-O's Extra Lean Turkey Bacon, cooked
- 2 oz 98% fat-free deli turkey
- 1 slice of fat-free cheddar cheese
- ¼ tsp Italian spice blend
- 2 tsps fat-free mayonnaise
- 2 slices of tomato
- Olive oil cooking spray

## Nutrition Information:

278 calories
32 g carbohydrates
5 g fiber
27 g protein
4 g fat
1 g saturated fat

## Directions

1. Spread each slice of bread with 1 tsp of mayonnaise.

2. Top one slice with turkey, bacon, and tomato. Top other slice with cheese, sprinkling with Italian seasoning, and close the sandwich.

3. Heat frying pan on medium heat. Spray lightly with cooking spray.

4. Place sandwich in pan, cheese side down, cooking for 2 minutes. Flip and cook an additional 1-2 minutes, until bread is toasted and cheese is melted.

# Seared Tilapia Salad

**Prep Time:** 10 minutes, **Total Time:** 15 minutes

This salad is packed with protein and B vitamins to keep you full and energized after lunch. The combination of spicy Dijon and sweet apples is sure to tantalize your taste buds.

## Directions

1. Heat frying pan over medium heat, spray lightly with olive oil cooking spray, and place tilapia filet in hot oil.

2. Season with dash of salt and pepper, and cook 2-3 minutes per side, or until done.

3. Set aside to let cool.

4. In a small bowl, mix together salad dressing ingredients: lime juice, mustard, olive oil, and a dash of salt and pepper.

5. Plate salad greens, and top with almonds, apple slices, and tilapia, broken into pieces. Drizzle with dressing and serve.

## Ingredients

- 2 cups mixed salad greens
- 1 6 oz tilapia filet, raw
- ½ tbsp lime juice
- 1 tsp honey Dijon mustard
- ½ tbsp olive oil
- ¼ apple, thinly sliced
- 1 tbsp sliced almonds
- Dash of salt and pepper
- Olive oil cooking spray

## Nutrition Information:

354 calories
11 g carbohydrates
3 g fiber
46 g protein
14 g fat
3 g saturated fat

# Tomato and Goat Cheese Mini Pizzas

**Prep Time:** 10 minutes, **Total Time:** 15 minutes

This colorful spin on pizza is a quick and easy end to a long day. It's also full of calcium and bursting with flavor.

## Ingredients

- 1 whole wheat English muffin
- 1 oz of crumbled goat cheese
- ¼ cup reduced fat mozzarella cheese
- ¼ tsp minced garlic
- ¼ cup chopped cherry tomatoes

## Directions

1. Cut English muffin in half.

2. Rub each half of the muffin with garlic.

3. Sprinkle with tomato and cheeses.

4. Broil in oven or toaster oven until cheese is melted. Serve and enjoy.

## Nutrition Information:

338 calories
30 g carbohydrates
5 g fiber, 22 g protein
16 g fat
10 g saturated fat

**Did You Know:**

Goat cheese is one of the earliest made dairy products, and comes in many shapes and flavors: cone-shaped, disc, wheel, strong and pungent, delicate and mild – the list is endless. Compared with cheese from a cow, goat cheese is lower in fat, calories, and cholesterol, and provides more calcium than cream cheese!

# Turkey Stuffed Bell Pepper

**Prep Time:** 30 minutes, **Total Time:** 1 hour & 30 minutes

This flavorful stuffed pepper is rich in B vitamins, potassium, vitamin C, and lean protein. Try making a larger batch of these for a quick and easy meal every night of the week.

## Directions

1. Preheat oven to 350°F.

2. In a skillet over medium-high heat, brown ground turkey.

3. Cut off the top stem part of bell pepper, removing seeds and membranes.

4. In a small bowl, mix together browned turkey, cooked rice, tomato sauce, Worcestershire sauce, garlic, onion powder, onion, and salt and pepper. Spoon mixture into hollowed out bell pepper.

5. Mix topping ingredients (Italian seasoning and ⅛ cup of tomato sauce) and pour over stuffed pepper.

6. Bake for 45 minutes to 1 hour in the oven, or until pepper is tender. Marinate occasionally with extra tomato sauce if desired.

## Ingredients

- 3 oz extra lean ground turkey, raw
- ¼ cup cooked brown rice
- 2 ½ tbsps water
- 1 green bell pepper
- ½ cup tomato sauce
- ½ tsp Worcestershire sauce
- ⅛ tsp minced garlic
- ⅛ tsp onion powder
- ¼ of 1 small white onion, diced
- Dash of salt and pepper

**Topping:**
- ⅛ tsp Italian seasoning
- ⅛ cup tomato sauce

## Nutrition Information:

255 calories, 28 g carbohydrates, 6 g fiber, 19 g protein, 8 g fat, 2 g saturated fat

# Eggplant Parmesan

**Prep Time:** 30 minutes, **Total Time:** 1 hour

This dish may taste and smell like comfort food, but the calorie-count says otherwise.

## Ingredients

- 1 slice of eggplant, about ¾ inch thick
- ½ tsp salt
- 1 tbsp olive oil
- 2 tbsps fat-free ricotta cheese
- 2 tbsps reduced-fat mozzarella cheese
- 1 tbsp fat-free parmesan cheese
- ⅛ cup egg substitutes (like Egg Beaters)
- 1 tsp dried basil
- ½ cup pasta sauce

## Nutrition Information:

321 calories
28 g carbohydrates
6 g fiber
15 g protein
17 g fat
4 g saturated fat

## Directions

1. Preheat oven to 350°F.

2. Sprinkle both sides of eggplant with salt, and let it sweat in a colander in the sink for 20-30 minutes.

3. While eggplant sweats, in a small bowl, mix together ricotta, mozzarella, parmesan cheese, egg, and dried basil. Set aside.

4. Heat frying pan on medium-high heat. Heat olive oil in pan.

5. Rinse the eggplant to remove salt, and transfer eggplant to pan. Brown each side of eggplant.

6. Pour pasta sauce into a small baking dish. Transfer eggplant slice on top of pasta sauce.

7. Top eggplant slice with cheese mixture.

8. Bake 30-45 minutes or until cheese bubbles.

# Lemon-Pepper Chicken and Rice

**Prep Time:** 5 minutes, **Total Time:** 8-10 hours

This refreshing chicken dish takes little prep work, and cooks for you while you bring home the monetary bacon. Throw these ingredients together in the morning and let it cook while you're at work for a delicious and simple meal when you walk through the door.

## Directions

1. Combine rice, water, and bouillon cube in crock pot.

2. Rub chicken breast with lemon peel, pepper, and sage, and place on top of rice. Sprinkle with minced garlic.

3. Let simmer for 8-10 hours, or until rice is fully cooked and water has been absorbed.

4. 10 minutes before serving, add frozen broccoli florets and sprinkle with salt and pepper. Let cook for 10 minutes to steam broccoli, then serve meal.

## Ingredients

- 1 3 oz chicken breast (raw)
- ¼ tsp lemon peel
- ¼ tsp ground black pepper
- ¼ tsp sage
- ½ tsp minced garlic
- ¼ cup brown rice, uncooked
- ½ bouillon cube
- ½ cup of water
- 1 cup of frozen broccoli florets
- Dash of salt and pepper

## Nutrition Information:

315 calories
45 g carbohydrates
7 g fiber
28 g protein
3 g fat
1 g saturated fat

# Sesame Seared Tuna with Wild Rice and Broccoli

**Prep Time:** 5 minutes, **Total Time:** 10 minutes

This dish combines the protein, vitamin D, and heart-healthy omega-3 fatty acids of tuna with the antioxidant-rich broccoli for winning flavor that's easy on your waistline.

## Ingredients:

- Olive oil cooking spray
- 1 3 oz tuna steak (any variety acceptable)
- ¼ cup low sodium soy sauce
- ½ tsp sesame oil
- 1 tbsp lemon juice
- ½ tsp ground ginger
- 2 tbsps sesame seeds
- ½ cup broccoli (fresh or frozen)
- ½ cup Uncle Ben's 90 second Ready Whole Grain Medley Brown and Wild Rice

## Nutrition Information:

405 calories
36 g carbohydrates
7 g fiber
32 g protein
16 g fat
2 g saturated fat

## Directions:

1. Place fry pan on burner at medium heat. Spritz lightly with olive oil spray and let heat thoroughly.

2. While burner heats, combine soy sauce, sesame oil, lemon juice, and ginger in a small, flat bottomed bowl.

3. Marinate tuna steak for 2 minutes on each side in sauce.

4. Coat each side of steak with sesame seeds, 1 tablespoon per side.

5. Once pan is heated, place tuna steak in pan, searing for 1 minute on each side.

6. While tuna is cooking, heat remainder of marinade in saucepan on stove. Once bubbling, remove from heat.

7. Set finished tuna aside and prepare rice according to directions. Plate ½ cup of rice with tuna, storing rest in refrigerator.

8. Place broccoli in a small dish with 1 tbsp of water, cover lightly, and microwave on high for 2 minutes. Sprinkle with pepper to taste.

9. Add broccoli to plate with tuna and rice. Pour remainder of heated marinade sauce over tuna and rice, and enjoy.

# Vegetarian Chili

**Prep Time: 10** minutes, Total Time: 6-8 minutes

The fabulous thing about this recipe is that it's minimal work with maximum flavor. Try combining the ingredients for this chili the night before and throwing them in your crock pot the next morning. You'll have a deliciously hot meal ready right when you get home! The bonus? This recipe makes TWO servings so you'll have another bowl ready for lunch the next day!

## Directions:

1. Combine all ingredients in small crock pot and let simmer for 6-8 hours.* Makes 2 servings.

   *Alternatively, you can combine ingredients in a saucepan and let simmer for 30 minutes on low heat before serving.

## Did You Know:

Texas-style chili contains no beans, and is often made with no other vegetables besides chili peppers. White chili is made using great northern beans and turkey meat or chicken breast. And lastly vegetarian chili, also known as chili "sin carne" (chili without meat), leaves meat out entirely or uses a meat analogue like tofu.

## Ingredients:

- 1 can of spicy chili beans
- 8 oz of salsa
- 1 8.75 oz can of whole kernel corn

## Nutrition Information:

1 serving of chili:
226 calories
43 g carbohydrates
11 g fiber
10 g protein
2 g fat
0 g saturated fat

# Spice Rubbed Salmon with Citrus Asparagus and Wild Rice

**Prep Time:** 10 minutes, **Total Time:** 30 minutes

If salmon seems like it's only a summer food, think again. This recipe warms up this classic summer dish, making even the coldest winter nights seem warm. Served with nutrient-rich asparagus, fiber-packed brown rice, and sweet and tangy onions, this meal is sure to please.

## Ingredients:
- Olive oil cooking spray
- ¼ white onion, sliced
- 7 asparagus spears (cut in half)
- 1 tsp lemon juice
- ½ tsp sea salt
- ⅛ tsp ground pepper
- ⅛ tsp ground coriander
- ¼ tsp paprika
- ¼ tsp ground cumin
- ½ cup Uncle Ben's 90 Second Ready Whole Grain Medley Brown and Wild Rice

## Nutrition Information:
329 calories
30 g carbohydrates,
5 g fiber
23 g protein
14 g fat
3 g saturated fat

## Directions
1. Preheat oven to 400°F.

2. Lightly coat 9x13 pan with cooking spray and fill with onion slices. Lay asparagus spears on top of onions and sprinkle them with the lemon juice. Spray both onions and asparagus lightly with olive oil spray.

3. Combine salt, pepper, coriander, paprika, and cumin in a small bowl. Rub mixture on salmon filet until well covered. Place salmon filet in pan on top of asparagus bed. Place pan in oven and bake for 20 minutes.

4. When salmon is close to being done, prepare rice according to directions. Plate ½ cup of rice, storing rest in refrigerator.

5. Remove pan from oven, place onions, asparagus, and salmon on top of rice, and enjoy!

# Black Bean and Spinach Quesadilla

**Prep Time:** 4 minutes, **Total Time:** 8 minutes

I love this recipe for adding a quick Mexican kick to dinner, sans the normal calorie-intake and fat load. This recipe makes a great dinner addition, but try making it the night before and it can also be a great re-heated lunch the next day.

## Directions

1. Heat burner to medium-high heat, and coat frying pan lightly with nonstick cooking spray.

2. Place tortilla flat in bottom of pan.

3. Add three slices of cheese to one half of quesadilla, top with spinach and beans, and sprinkle on taco seasoning.

4. Cook until cheese is melted, or until tortilla is crisp.

5. When cheese is fully melted, use a spatula to flip other half of tortilla over to close the quesadilla, and pat together to close it. Flip once more to cook lightly on other side.

6. Once cheese is fully melted, remove from pan and serve with salsa.

## Ingredients

- 1 La Tortilla Factory 100% Whole Wheat 100 Calorie Tortilla
- ½ cup frozen spinach, thawed
- ⅛ cup canned black bean, rinsed to remove excess salt
- 3 slices of fat-free white American cheese
- ¼ tsp taco seasoning
- Cooking spray
- ¼ cup salsa

## Nutrition Information:

265 calories
45 g carbohydrates
13 g fiber
25 g protein
3 g fat
0 g saturated fat

# Baked Spaghetti Pie

**Prep Time:** 13 minutes, **Total Time:** 40 minutes

Bored with plain spaghetti? Mix it up with this quick and easy spaghetti pie – a low-calorie twist on an Italian classic.

## Ingredients

- ¾ cup cooked spaghetti noodles
- ¼ cup Egg Beaters
- ¼ tsp oregano leaves
- ¼ tsp ground pepper
- ⅛ cup fat-free ricotta cheese
- 2 tbsp fat-free parmesan cheese
- ⅓ cup marinara sauce
- Olive oil cooking spray

## Nutrition Information:

362 calories
54 g carbohydrates
8 g fiber
27 g protein
4 g fat
2 g saturated fat

## Directions

1. Preheat oven to 350°F.

2. Stir egg beaters, parmesan cheese, oregano, and black pepper in with cooked spaghetti noodles.

3. Spray an oven-safe ramekin or a small, single serving casserole bowl with cooking spray.

4. Place noodles in bowl and top with ricotta cheese, followed by marinara sauce. Bake for 20 minutes.

5. Remove from oven and let cool for 7 minutes before serving.

# Spicy Chipotle Chicken

**Prep Time:** 3 minutes, **Total Time:** 5-6 hours

This slow-cooked chicken meal is low in saturated fat, a good source of fiber, and a fantastic way to get your protein. Plus it's packed with flavors that will make your taste buds curl.

## Directions

1. Place chicken breast in bottom of a crock pot and surround with salsa.

2. Sprinkle chicken with cumin, chipotle chile pepper, chili powder, and minced garlic.

3. Top with black beans.

4. Let simmer for 5-6 hours, or until chicken is thoroughly cooked.

5. 10 minutes before serving, add bell pepper mix. Let cook until bell peppers are thoroughly cooked and serve.

## Ingredients

- 1 3 oz skinless, boneless chicken breast (raw)
- ⅛ cup salsa
- ¼ tsp ground cumin
- ¼ tsp chipotle chile pepper
- ⅛ tsp chili powder
- 1 clove of minced garlic
- ¼ 15.5 oz can black beans (rinsed to remove excess sodium)
- 1 cup frozen bell pepper mix

## Nutrition Information:

278 calories
34 g carbohydrates
11 g fiber
31 g protein
2 g fat
0 g saturated fat

# Black Pepper Tuna With Artichokes and Tomatoes

**Prep Time:** 10 minutes, **Total Time:** 20 minutes

Tuna is full of heart-healthy omega-3 fatty acids. The artichoke hearts in this dish provide a winning flavor that's easy on your waistline and extraordinary on your taste buds.

## Ingredients

- ¾ cup frozen artichoke hearts, thawed
- 3 tbsps diced, canned tomatoes
- 1 ½ tsp olive oil
- 1 clove minced garlic
- ½ tbsp lemon juice
- ¼ tsp ground thyme
- 1 6 oz Ahi tuna steak, raw
- ½ cup brown rice, cooked (recommended: 90 second rice)
- Dash of salt and pepper
- Olive oil cooking spray

## Nutrition Information:

395 calories
32 g carbohydrates
5 g fiber
45 g protein
9 g fat
2 g saturated fat

## Directions

1. Prepare brown rice according to directions, plate ½ cup and set aside.

2. Place fry pan on burner on medium heat. Let it heat thoroughly, and spritz lightly with olive oil spray.

3. While burner heats, combine artichoke hearts, tomatoes, olive oil, garlic, lemon juice, and thyme in a frying pan and stir over medium heat.

4. Sprinkle each side of tuna steak lightly with salt and pepper.

5. Once pan is heated, place tuna steak in pan, searing for 1 minute on each side.

6. While tuna is cooking, continue to stir artichoke and tomato mixture. Sprinkle with a dash of salt and pepper.

7. Set finished tuna on top of rice.

8. Transfer artichoke and tomato mixture from pan onto tuna and rice.

# Black Bean Soup

**Prep Time:** 2 minutes, **Total Time:** 18 minutes

Homemade soup is the perfect way to warm up on a chilly day, or even just to give you a little bit of comfort. This recipe is great for both, and is packed with nutrient-rich beans, fiber, and protein. Want leftovers? Simply double the recipe and you'll have some for lunch tomorrow!

## Directions

1. Heat olive oil over medium heat in a saucepan. Add ⅓ cup salsa and cook for 2-3 minutes.

2. Add in black beans, refried beans, and vegetable broth, bringing to a boil. Reduce heat and simmer for 5 minutes.

3. Pour soup into a bowl and top with sour cream, 1 tbsp of salsa, and cilantro. Serve.

**Did You Know:**

Research has shown that draining and rinsing your canned beans can reduce sodium by up to 40%! The USDA's Dietary Guidelines recommends the general U.S. population limit their sodium intake to less than a teaspoon.

## Ingredients

**Soup:**
- ¼ tsp olive oil
- ⅓ cup salsa
- ½ cup canned black beans, rinsed to remove excess sodium
- ½ cup fat-free refried beans
- ½ cup low-sodium vegetable broth

**Topping:**
- 1 tbsp fat-free sour cream
- 1 tbsp salsa
- 1 tbsp freshly chopped cilantro

**Nutrition Information:**
263 calories
46 g carbohydrates
14 g fiber
16 g protein
2 g fat
0 g saturated fat

# Penne and Green Bean Pasta Salad

**Prep Time:** 15 minutes, **Total Time:** 20 minutes

Pack your lunch with fiber and vitamins this week with this simple pasta salad. Make it the night before and you'll be ready to rush out the door in the morning, confident that you'll have a delicious lunch ready come noon.

## Ingredients

- ¾ cup cooked, whole wheat penne pasta noodles, cooled
- ½ cup halved green beans, steamed
- ¼ cup canned kidney beans, rinsed to remove excess sodium
- 1 tbsp parsley
- 1 tbsp fat-free parmesan cheese
- 2 tsps olive oil
- 1 tbsp lemon juice
- Salt and pepper to taste

## Nutrition Information:
365 calories
53 g carbohydrates
10 g fiber
16 g protein
12 g fat
2 g saturated fat

## Directions

1. Toss together cooked noodles, steamed green beans, and kidney beans. Add in parsley, parmesan, olive oil, lemon juice, and ¼ tsp of salt and pepper each. Mix thoroughly.

2. Refrigerate overnight and serve.

**Did You Know:**
With its mild flavor, fresh chopped parsley is often used as a garnish, frequently topping chicken soups, green salads, and cold cuts. It is also commonly believed that chewing parsley can counteract the bad breath effects of garlic after a meal.

# Pan Seared Tilapia and Clementine Salad

**Prep Time:** 6 minutes, **Total Time:** 15 minutes

This fish dish is packed with protein, spices, and vitamins, and is sure to delight even the most discriminating of taste-buds.

## Directions

1. Heat frying pan on medium-high heat. Spray lightly with olive oil cooking spray.

2. Season tilapia fillet with salt and pepper, and add to pan.

3. Cook 1-2 minutes on each side, or until it's cooked through and easily flakes. Transfer to plate.

4. In a small container with a lid, mix together olive oil, lime juice, ginger, honey, salt, and red pepper.

5. Plate salad greens and top with Clementine orange slices. Plate fish with salad.

6. Drizzle fish and salad with dressing and serve.

## Ingredients

- 1 3 oz fillet of tilapia, raw
- Dash of salt and ground black pepper
- 1 Clementine orange, peeled and sectioned
- 1 cup mixed salad greens
- Olive oil cooking spray

**Dressing:**
- 1 tbsp olive oil
- ½ tbsp lime juice
- ½ tsp crushed ginger
- ½ tsp honey
- ⅛ tsp salt
- Dash of crushed red pepper

## Nutrition Information:
283 calories
14 g carbohydrates
2 g fiber
23 g protein
16 g fat
3 g saturated fat

# White Bean Chicken and Tomatoes

**Prep Time:** 5 minutes, **Total Time:** 30 minutes

You won't be disappointed as the aroma of thyme and oregano fill your kitchen with this simple and delicious recipe. And your stomach will be thanking you when it gets the 33 grams of satisfying protein and 10 grams of filling fiber.

## Ingredients

- 1 3 oz boneless, skinless, chicken breast (raw)
- ¾ cup white beans, rinsed to remove excess sodium
- ½ cup cherry tomatoes, cut in half
- 1 tsp thyme
- 1 tsp oregano
- ½ clove minced garlic
- ⅛ tsp crushed red pepper
- 1 ½ tsps olive oil
- ⅛ tsp salt
- ⅛ tsp ground black pepper

## Nutrition Information:

352 calories
37 g carbohydrates
10 g fiber
33 g protein
8 g fat
1 g saturated fat

## Directions

1. Preheat oven to 425°F.

2. Combine beans, tomatoes, thyme, oregano, minced garlic, red pepper, 1 tsp olive oil, salt, and pepper in a small baking dish.

3. Place chicken breast on top of bean mixture and rub with remaining ½ tsp olive oil. Season lightly with dash of salt and pepper.

4. Bake dish until chicken is cooked thoroughly, about 25-30 minutes.

# Cilantro-Lime Chicken and Salsa

**Prep Time:** 20 minutes, **Total Time:** 30 minutes

The aroma of cilantro will fill the air, and the tangy taste of lime will be biting at your tongue when you whip up this delicious chicken dish.

## Directions

1. In a small bowl, mix cilantro, lime juice, olive oil, and salt. Marinate chicken in mixture for 3-5 minutes.

2. Heat frying pan over medium-high heat. Spray lightly with cooking spray and when heated, transfer chicken into pan. Top with a few tablespoons of marinade, and cook for 5-6 minutes on each side, or until completely cooked.

3. In a separate bowl, combine ingredients for salsa: tomatoes, onion, avocado, lime juice, garlic, and salt and pepper, mixing thoroughly.

4. Plate chicken on top of rice, and pour salsa over both.

## Ingredients

- 1 4 oz boneless, skinless, chicken breast (raw)
- ½ cup brown rice, cooked
- ½ tbsp minced cilantro
- 1 ¾ tsps lime juice
- 1 ⅛ tsps olive oil
- Dash of salt
- Olive oil cooking spray

**Salsa:**

- ¼ cup cherry tomatoes, chopped
- ½ tbsp chopped red onion
- ¼ avocado, peeled, pitted, and chopped
- ½ tsp lime juice
- ⅛ tsp minced garlic
- Dash of salt and pepper

## Nutrition Information:

346 calories, 28 g carbohydrates, 5 g fiber, 30 g protein, 13 g fat, 2 g saturated fat

# Penne Pasta e Fagioli

**Prep Time:** 15 minutes, **Total Time:** 20 minutes

Pasta e fagioli means "pasta and beans" in Italian. It may sound boring, but this dish is anything but. The beans pack a lot of fiber, and combined with the colorful tomato, as well as the flavorful oregano, you'll almost feel like you're sitting in Venice.

## Ingredients

- 1 cup cooked, whole wheat penne pasta noodles
- ½ tsp olive oil
- 1 clove garlic, minced
- ⅓ cup canned white beans, rinsed to remove excess sodium
- ½ cup diced tomato
- 1 tbsp fat-free parmesan cheese
- ½ tsp oregano
- Salt and pepper to taste

## Nutrition Information:

375 calories
66 g carbohydrates
11 g fiber
19 g protein
5 g fat
1 g saturated fat

## Directions

1. Heat frying pan on medium heat and combine olive oil, tomato, garlic, and beans.

2. When bean mixture is thoroughly heated, remove from frying pan and add to small bowl with cooked penne pasta noodles.

3. Add parmesan cheese and oregano, stir, and serve.

### Did You Know:

Garlic has been used for both culinary and medicinal purposes throughout the years, and was even mentioned in the Bible. Crushing or cutting garlic releases a compound called allicin, which research has shown may aid in heart health.

# Sweet & Savory Meatless Tacos

**Prep Time:** 15 minutes, **Total Time:** 20 minutes

Meatless taco night doesn't have to mean just beans – Morningstar Farms' delicious meatless-meat crumbles are the perfect substitution in tacos. Low in fat, the crumbles are packed in protein, and the mango salsa on these tacos packs a sweet tang to offset the zesty kick of taco seasoning.

## Directions

1. Heat frying pan on medium-high heat. Pour in frozen Morningstar crumbles, water, and taco seasoning. Heat, stirring until heated thoroughly.

2. Split taco meat evenly between tortillas.

3. Top each taco with 2 tbsps of salsa, 2 tbsps sour cream, ½ cup lettuce, and ¼ cup diced tomatoes.

4. Roll and serve.

## Ingredients

- 2 La Tortilla Factory 100% Whole Wheat 50 Calorie Tortillas
- 1 cup frozen Morningstar Farms Meal Starters Grillers Recipe Crumbles
- ½ packet of taco seasoning
- ⅓ cup of water
- 4 tbsps Newman's Own Mango Salsa
- 4 tbsps fat-free sour cream
- 1 cup shredded romaine lettuce
- ½ cup diced tomatoes

## Nutrition Information:

323 calories, 57 g carbohydrates, 18 g fiber, 24 g protein, 5 g fat, 0 g saturated fat

# Garlic & Lemon Shrimp and Couscous

**Prep Time:** 15 minutes, **Total Time:** 25 minutes

The couscous in this dish brings a hint of exotic flavor, but is super easy to prepare, and is a great source of filling fiber and protein.

## Ingredients

- ⅓ cup couscous, cooked
- ½ tbsp butter
- ½ clove minced garlic
- 4 oz shrimp, cooked, peeled, and deveined
- ½ cup canned white beans, rinsed to remove excess sodium
- ½ tbsp lemon juice
- 1 tbsp parsley
- ⅛ tsp salt
- ⅛ tsp pepper

## Nutrition Information:
345 calories
36 g carbohydrates
10 g fiber
32 g protein
7 g fat
2 g saturated fat

## Directions

1. Cook couscous according to package directions. Set aside ⅓ up for meal, store rest in refrigerator.

2. Heat butter in frying pan on medium heat.

3. Add garlic and shrimp, and heat for about 3-4 minutes, or until thoroughly cooked through.

4. Stir in beans, lemon juice, parsley, salt, and pepper.

5. Cook until thoroughly heated, serve shrimp mixture over couscous.

# Red Bean & Rice Burrito

**Prep Time:** 6 minutes, **Total Time:** 12 minutes

Cilantro and spinach really spice up this low-calorie burrito, and the beans and whole wheat tortilla also make it a great source of filling fiber.

## Directions

1. Sauté onion in olive oil over medium heat for roughly 3 minutes.

2. Add rice, beans, salt, and cilantro, and cook for another 2 minutes.

3. Put bean and rice mixture in tortilla and top with spinach, cheese, salsa, and sour cream.

4. Roll into a burrito and enjoy.

## Ingredients

- 1 La Tortilla Factory 100% Whole Wheat 100 Calorie Tortilla
- 2 tbsps chopped onion
- 1 tsp olive oil
- ⅛ tsp salt
- ¼ brown rice, cooked
- ¼ cup canned pinto beans, rinsed to remove excess sodium
- 1 tbsp cilantro
- 2 tbsps shredded low-fat Monterey Jack cheese
- ½ cup fresh baby spinach leaves
- 2 tbsps salsa
- 2 tbsps fat-free sour cream

## Nutrition Information:
346 calories
56 g carbohydrates
14 g fiber
16 g protein
10 g fat
3 g saturated fat

# 20 Healthy Snacks Under 200 Calories

1. 2 tbsps peanut butter
   15 whole wheat crackers

2. Baby carrots, red peppers
   2 tbsps hummus

3. Laughing Cow Light Cheese
   15 whole wheat crackers

4. Sliced papaya with lime juice

5. Low-fat string cheese
   Apple or pear

6. Can of tuna
   Sliced black olives
   Lemon juice

7. Peanut butter
   Apple

8. Multi-grain pita
   2 tbsps hummus

9. Sliced tomato
   Sliced mozzarella
   Drizzle of olive oil

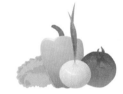

**Did You Know:**
The USDA says you should eat 3-5 servings of vegetables a day.

10. 1 oz raspberries
    Cottage cheese

11. 2 slices of turkey
    1 slice Swiss or American cheese
    Mustard for dipping

12. 4 cups light popcorn (25 calories per cup)
    Sprinkle of parmesan cheese

13. 1 cup raspberries
    20-25 almonds

14. 5 strawberries
    Cool Whip Light

15. 1 tbsp almond butter
    Apple

16. 2 slices of turkey
    Small multi-grain tortilla
    Salsa

17. ½ cup cottage cheese
    20-25 almonds

18. 5-10 olives
    1 cup unshelled edamame

19. Cottage cheese
    Canned pineapple, drained

20. 1 cup sugar snap peas
    2 tbsps parmesan cheese

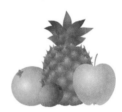

**Did You Know:**
Sometimes the time of day is enough encouragement to eat a meal, despite a lack of actual physical hunger. But don't eat a big meal just because it's lunch time. Instead, learn to listen to your body. A quick snack may be all you need.

# Chapter 17

"When the grass looks greener on the other side of the fence, it may be that they take better care of it there."
~ Unknown

# How to Use the Journal Pages

These journal pages are an instrumental part of losing weight fast because they help you monitor your weight, calorie intake, and calories burned through exercise. The best way to create a significant calorie deficit every day is to plan ahead. Create a calorie "budget" for each meal and snack, and determine how much exercise you need to burn additional calories. Anticipating how many calories you can "spend" at each meal takes the guesswork out of cooking and ordering off restaurant menus. For instance, if you have 400 calories to budget for lunch, you may decide to order a turkey sub with cheese and spend the whole amount, or you may opt for the veggie sub with no cheese and save 150 calories.

The journal pages also give you clues into how food, exercise and hydration factor into your mood and energy levels. You may find fascinating correlations between what and when you're eating, and how great or lousy you're feeling. Plus, nothing is a better motivator for exercise than realizing how much more energy and stamina you have throughout the day after you've hit the gym or gone for a bike ride.

Another great benefit of a diet and fitness journal is it keeps you accountable. It's easy to let a 150-calorie cookie slip your mind, or to tell yourself you worked out for 30 minutes when it was really only 20, but those little white lies are much more difficult when you're recording everything in a journal throughout the day. You've likely put on extra weight by not holding yourself accountable in the past; this journal will help you break that bad habit and start keeping track of everything you eat, drink, and do by way of exercise. It's the proven way to slim down faster!

Here is an explanation of the different components of the journal pages:

**❶ DAILY NUTRITIONAL INTAKE:** Record your daily intake of calories, fats and carbs for each meal and snack. Write down your totals for breakfast, lunch, dinner, and 2 snacks. Compare these totals to your nutritional intake goal from earlier in this book and see if you are meeting or going over your target amounts. There is also a column called "Other" that can be used to track intake of protein, fiber, sugar, sodium or another nutrient if you have special dietary concerns, such as high blood pressure or diabetes.

**❷ WATER INTAKE:** Strive for at least eight 8-ounce glasses of water per day. Check off a box for each glass you drink. If you drink water on a regular basis throughout the day, your metabolism works faster and better and you'll have more energy for exercise.

**❸ DAILY NUMBER OF SERVINGS:** At the end of each day, write down the number of servings you ate from each of the 6 major food groups. Eating a balanced diet is a big part of losing weight and keeping it off.

**❹ VITAMINS & SUPPLEMENTS:** Make note of the vitamins or supplements you are including in your program. When in doubt about specific vitamin recommendations, consult with a health care professional.

**❺ DAILY GOAL:** Write down a goal each day and try your best to stick to it. When you do meet your daily goal, check off the box and you can feel proud of your success!

**❻ PHYSICAL ACTIVITY:** Record all physical activity you perform, including cardio, strength training, flexibility training, or a combination of all 3. Record the duration, distance, pace, weight, sets, number of repetitions, and total calories burned.

**❼ CALORIE CALCULATOR:** This formula helps you find your Daily Net Calorie Gain or Loss for each day. Start with your Total Calorie Intake for that day, subtract the Total Calories Burned from physical activity to get Net Calories. Then, subtract your BMR (the number of calories your body burns at rest, calculated earlier in this book) to get your Daily Net Calorie Gain or Loss. Your goal is for this to be a negative number, meaning you created a calorie deficit, which is necessary to lose weight.

**❽ ENERGY LEVEL:** Document your daily overall energy by rating your energy levels from 1 to 6. Take note of how your energy correlates to the types of foods you have eaten that day. For example, if you notice that a little extra protein helps you get through your workout with more energy, incorporate lean meats in your diet. As you discover these relationships, make adjustments as needed to help you feel your best.

**❾ MUSCLE GROUP WORKED:** Document which of the 6 major muscle groups you work each day during exercise. Strive to include workouts that work your entire body, but also pay attention to how your body feels and give certain muscle groups sufficient rest to prevent injury.

## Sample Journal Page

# DIET JOURNAL

# Day 1

DATE: Feb. 2          WEIGHT: 197

### ❶ BREAKFAST

| BREAKFAST | Qty. | Calories | Fat | Carbs | Protein Other |
|---|---|---|---|---|---|
| Blueberry scone | 1 | 400 | 17 | 55 | 5 |
| Orange juice | 12 oz. | 110 | 0 | 26 | 2 |
| | | | | | |
| | | | | | |
| | | | | | |

| SNACK | Qty. | Calories | Fat | Carbs | Other |
|---|---|---|---|---|---|
| | | | | | |
| | | | | | |

| LUNCH | Qty. | Calories | Fat | Carbs | Other |
|---|---|---|---|---|---|
| Bagel w/turkey | | 490 | 4 | 70 | 30 |
| American cheese | 2 | 64 | 2 | 2 | 8 |
| Baby carrots | | 100 | 0 | 24 | 3 |
| Pepsi | 12 oz. | 180 | 0 | 45 | 0 |
| | | | | | |

| SNACK | Qty. | Calories | Fat | Carbs | Other |
|---|---|---|---|---|---|
| Apple slices and peanut butter | | 245 | 17 | 21 | 10 |

| DINNER | Qty. | Calories | Fat | Carbs | Other |
|---|---|---|---|---|---|
| Salmon | 8 oz. | 416 | 22 | 0 | 45 |
| Wild rice | | 166 | 2 | 34 | 7 |
| Broccoli | | 54 | 1 | 12 | 2 |
| Crystal Light Tea | | 5 | 0 | 0 | 0 |
| | | | | | |
| **DAILY INTAKE TOTALS:** | | 2,230 | 65 | 289 | 112 |

❷ ☑ Water Intake
# of 8 oz. glasses
✓ ✓ ✓
✓ ✓ ✓
✓ ✓ ☐

❸ Daily # of Servings
3 fruits    2 meats & beans
2 veggies   1 milk & dairy
3 grains    3 oils & sweets

❹ Vitamins & Supplements:
Calcium
Vitamin C

# FITNESS JOURNAL

**⑤**

**DAILY GOAL:** Eat a high protein dinner + work out for 90⁺ mins.   **GOAL MET:** ☑

### 🏃 CARDIOVASCULAR EXERCISE   **⑥**

| Exercise | Duration | Distance | Pace | Cal. Burned |
|---|---|---|---|---|
| Shooting the basketball | 60 mins | | medium | 300 |
| Jogging around my neighborhood | 20 mins | 1.5 mi | 4.5mph | 205 |
| | | | | |
| | | | | |

### 🏋 STRENGTH TRAINING

| Exercise | Weight | Reps. | Sets | Cal. Burned |
|---|---|---|---|---|
| Bicep curls | 25 | 3 | 36 | 20 |
| Pull-ups | | 2 | 8 | 25 |
| Push-ups | | 2 | 60 | 35 |
| | | | | |
| | | | | |
| | | | | |
| | | | | |

### 🧘 FLEXIBILITY, RELAXATION, MEDITATION

| Activity | Duration | Cal. Burned |
|---|---|---|
| Stretching | 10 mins | 5 |
| | | |
| | | |
| | | |

**DAILY CALORIES BURNED:** 590

**⑦**

### CALORIE CALCULATOR

| 2,230 | − | 590 | = | 1,640 | − | 1,979 | = | −339 |
|---|---|---|---|---|---|---|---|---|
| TOTAL CALORIE INTAKE | | TOTAL CALORIES BURNED | | NET CALORIES | | BMR (Basal Metabolic Rate) | | DAILY NET CALORIE GAIN OR LOSS |

**⑧** 👎 **Energy Level:** 1  2  3  4  ⑤  6 👍

**⑨** **Muscle Group Worked:** ☑arms ☑chest ☐back ☐core ☑thighs ☑calves

**Diet & Workout Notes:**
Need more fiber during breakfast! Buy oatmeal. Do 45 minutes of cardio tomorrow.

# DIET JOURNAL

# Day 1

DATE:_____     WEIGHT:_____

| BREAKFAST | Qty. | Calories | Fat | Carbs | Other |
|-----------|------|----------|-----|-------|-------|
| | | | | | |
| | | | | | |
| | | | | | |
| | | | | | |
| | | | | | |

| SNACK | Qty. | Calories | Fat | Carbs | Other |
|-------|------|----------|-----|-------|-------|
| | | | | | |
| | | | | | |

| LUNCH | Qty. | Calories | Fat | Carbs | Other |
|-------|------|----------|-----|-------|-------|
| | | | | | |
| | | | | | |
| | | | | | |
| | | | | | |
| | | | | | |

| SNACK | Qty. | Calories | Fat | Carbs | Other |
|-------|------|----------|-----|-------|-------|
| | | | | | |
| | | | | | |

| DINNER | Qty. | Calories | Fat | Carbs | Other |
|--------|------|----------|-----|-------|-------|
| | | | | | |
| | | | | | |
| | | | | | |
| | | | | | |
| | | | | | |

**DAILY INTAKE TOTALS:**

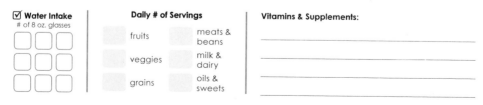

☑ **Water Intake**
# of 8 oz. glasses

**Daily # of Servings**

- fruits
- veggies
- grains
- meats & beans
- milk & dairy
- oils & sweets

**Vitamins & Supplements:**

_____
_____
_____
_____

# FITNESS JOURNAL

DAILY GOAL: _____ GOAL MET: ☐

### 🏃 CARDIOVASCULAR EXERCISE

| | Duration | Distance | Pace | Cal. Burned |
|---|---|---|---|---|
| | | | | |
| | | | | |
| | | | | |
| | | | | |

### 🏋 STRENGTH TRAINING

| | Weight | Reps. | Sets | Cal. Burned |
|---|---|---|---|---|
| | | | | |
| | | | | |
| | | | | |
| | | | | |
| | | | | |
| | | | | |
| | | | | |
| | | | | |

### 大 FLEXIBILITY, RELAXATION, MEDITATION

| | Duration | Cal. Burned |
|---|---|---|
| | | |
| | | |
| | | |

**DAILY CALORIES BURNED:** _____

---

### CALORIE CALCULATOR

| _____ | − | _____ | = | _____ | − | _____ | = | _____ |
|---|---|---|---|---|---|---|---|---|
| TOTAL CALORIE INTAKE | | TOTAL CALORIES BURNED | | NET CALORIES | | BMR (Basal Metabolic Rate) | | DAILY NET CALORIE GAIN OR LOSS |

**Energy Level:** 👎 1  2  3  4  5  6 👍

**Muscle Group Worked:** ☐ arms ☐ chest ☐ back ☐ core ☐ thighs ☐ calves

**Diet & Workout Notes:**

_____

_____

_____

_____

# Day 2

DATE: _____          WEIGHT: _____

🍎 **BREAKFAST** _____

| | Qty. | Calories | Fat | Carbs | Other |
|---|---|---|---|---|---|
| _____ | ____ | | | | |
| _____ | ____ | | | | |
| _____ | ____ | | | | |
| _____ | ____ | | | | |
| _____ | ____ | | | | |

➕ **SNACK** _____

| | Qty. | Calories | Fat | Carbs | Other |
|---|---|---|---|---|---|
| _____ | ____ | | | | |
| _____ | ____ | | | | |

🍽 **LUNCH** _____

| | Qty. | Calories | Fat | Carbs | Other |
|---|---|---|---|---|---|
| _____ | ____ | | | | |
| _____ | ____ | | | | |
| _____ | ____ | | | | |
| _____ | ____ | | | | |
| _____ | ____ | | | | |

🍇 **SNACK** _____

| | Qty. | Calories | Fat | Carbs | Other |
|---|---|---|---|---|---|
| _____ | ____ | | | | |
| _____ | ____ | | | | |

🍴 **DINNER** _____

| | Qty. | Calories | Fat | Carbs | Other |
|---|---|---|---|---|---|
| _____ | ____ | | | | |
| _____ | ____ | | | | |
| _____ | ____ | | | | |
| _____ | ____ | | | | |
| _____ | ____ | | | | |

**DAILY INTAKE TOTALS:**

☑ **Water Intake**
# of 8 oz. glasses

☐ ☐ ☐
☐ ☐ ☐
☐ ☐ ☐

**Daily # of Servings**

fruits          meats & beans

veggies        milk & dairy

grains         oils & sweets

**Vitamins & Supplements:**

_____

_____

_____

_____

# FITNESS JOURNAL

DAILY GOAL: _____     GOAL MET: ☐

### 🏃 CARDIOVASCULAR EXERCISE

| | Duration | Distance | Pace | Cal. Burned |
|---|---|---|---|---|
| _____ | | | | |
| _____ | | | | |
| _____ | | | | |
| _____ | | | | |

### 🏋 STRENGTH TRAINING

| | Weight | Reps. | Sets | Cal. Burned |
|---|---|---|---|---|
| _____ | | | | |
| _____ | | | | |
| _____ | | | | |
| _____ | | | | |
| _____ | | | | |
| _____ | | | | |
| _____ | | | | |
| _____ | | | | |

### 🧘 FLEXIBILITY, RELAXATION, MEDITATION

| | Duration | Cal. Burned |
|---|---|---|
| _____ | | |
| _____ | | |
| _____ | | |

**DAILY CALORIES BURNED:** ____

---

## CALORIE CALCULATOR

| ____ | − | ____ | = | ____ | − | ____ | = | ____ |
|---|---|---|---|---|---|---|---|---|
| TOTAL CALORIE INTAKE | | TOTAL CALORIES BURNED | | NET CALORIES | | BMR (Basal Metabolic Rate) | | DAILY NET CALORIE GAIN OR LOSS |

---

**Energy Level:**   👎  1  2  3  4  5  6  👍

**Muscle Group Worked:**  ☐ arms  ☐ chest  ☐ back  ☐ core  ☐ thighs  ☐ calves

**Diet & Workout Notes:**

_____

_____

_____

_____

# Day 3

DATE: _____     WEIGHT: _____

| 🍎 BREAKFAST | Qty. | Calories | Fat | Carbs | Other |
|---|---|---|---|---|---|
| _____ | _____ | | | | |
| _____ | _____ | | | | |
| _____ | _____ | | | | |
| _____ | _____ | | | | |
| _____ | _____ | | | | |

| 🥛 SNACK | Qty. | Calories | Fat | Carbs | Other |
|---|---|---|---|---|---|
| _____ | _____ | | | | |
| _____ | _____ | | | | |

| 🍱 LUNCH | Qty. | Calories | Fat | Carbs | Other |
|---|---|---|---|---|---|
| _____ | _____ | | | | |
| _____ | _____ | | | | |
| _____ | _____ | | | | |
| _____ | _____ | | | | |
| _____ | _____ | | | | |

| 🍇 SNACK | Qty. | Calories | Fat | Carbs | Other |
|---|---|---|---|---|---|
| _____ | _____ | | | | |
| _____ | _____ | | | | |

| 🍳 DINNER | Qty. | Calories | Fat | Carbs | Other |
|---|---|---|---|---|---|
| _____ | _____ | | | | |
| _____ | _____ | | | | |
| _____ | _____ | | | | |
| _____ | _____ | | | | |
| _____ | _____ | | | | |

**DAILY INTAKE TOTALS:**

☑ **Water Intake**
# of 8 oz. glasses

☐ ☐ ☐
☐ ☐ ☐
☐ ☐ ☐

**Daily # of Servings**

| | |
|---|---|
| fruits | meats & beans |
| veggies | milk & dairy |
| grains | oils & sweets |

**Vitamins & Supplements:**

_____
_____
_____
_____

# FITNESS JOURNAL

DAILY GOAL: _____     GOAL MET: ☐

### 🏃 CARDIOVASCULAR EXERCISE

| | Duration | Distance | Pace | Cal. Burned |
|---|---|---|---|---|
| _____ | | | | |
| _____ | | | | |
| _____ | | | | |
| _____ | | | | |

### 🏋 STRENGTH TRAINING

| | Weight | Reps. | Sets | Cal. Burned |
|---|---|---|---|---|
| _____ | | | | |
| _____ | | | | |
| _____ | | | | |
| _____ | | | | |
| _____ | | | | |
| _____ | | | | |
| _____ | | | | |

### 🧘 FLEXIBILITY, RELAXATION, MEDITATION

| | Duration | Cal. Burned |
|---|---|---|
| _____ | | |
| _____ | | |
| _____ | | |

**DAILY CALORIES BURNED:** _____

## CALORIE CALCULATOR

| ___ | − | ___ | = | ___ | − | ___ | = | ___ |
|---|---|---|---|---|---|---|---|---|
| TOTAL CALORIE INTAKE | | TOTAL CALORIES BURNED | | NET CALORIES | | BMR (Basal Metabolic Rate) | | DAILY NET CALORIE GAIN OR LOSS |

**Energy Level:**  👎  1  2  3  4  5  6  👍

**Muscle Group Worked:** ☐ arms ☐ chest ☐ back ☐ core ☐ thighs ☐ calves

**Diet & Workout Notes:**

_____

_____

_____

_____

# Day 4

DATE: _____     WEIGHT: _____

## 🍎 BREAKFAST

| | Qty. | Calories | Fat | Carbs | Other |
|---|---|---|---|---|---|
| _____ | _____ | | | | |
| _____ | _____ | | | | |
| _____ | _____ | | | | |
| _____ | _____ | | | | |
| _____ | _____ | | | | |

## SNACK

| | Qty. | Calories | Fat | Carbs | Other |
|---|---|---|---|---|---|
| _____ | _____ | | | | |
| _____ | _____ | | | | |

## LUNCH

| | Qty. | Calories | Fat | Carbs | Other |
|---|---|---|---|---|---|
| _____ | _____ | | | | |
| _____ | _____ | | | | |
| _____ | _____ | | | | |
| _____ | _____ | | | | |
| _____ | _____ | | | | |

## SNACK

| | Qty. | Calories | Fat | Carbs | Other |
|---|---|---|---|---|---|
| _____ | _____ | | | | |
| _____ | _____ | | | | |

## DINNER

| | Qty. | Calories | Fat | Carbs | Other |
|---|---|---|---|---|---|
| _____ | _____ | | | | |
| _____ | _____ | | | | |
| _____ | _____ | | | | |
| _____ | _____ | | | | |
| _____ | _____ | | | | |

**DAILY INTAKE TOTALS:**

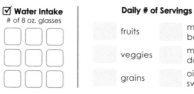

☑ **Water Intake**
# of 8 oz. glasses

**Daily # of Servings**

| | |
|---|---|
| fruits | meats & beans |
| veggies | milk & dairy |
| grains | oils & sweets |

**Vitamins & Supplements:**

_____
_____
_____
_____

# FITNESS JOURNAL

DAILY GOAL: _____   GOAL MET: ☐

### 🏃 CARDIOVASCULAR EXERCISE

| | Duration | Distance | Pace | Cal. Burned |
|---|---|---|---|---|
| _____ | | | | |
| _____ | | | | |
| _____ | | | | |
| _____ | | | | |

### 🏋 STRENGTH TRAINING

| | Weight | Reps. | Sets | Cal. Burned |
|---|---|---|---|---|
| _____ | | | | |
| _____ | | | | |
| _____ | | | | |
| _____ | | | | |
| _____ | | | | |
| _____ | | | | |
| _____ | | | | |
| _____ | | | | |

### 方 FLEXIBILITY, RELAXATION, MEDITATION

| | Duration | Cal. Burned |
|---|---|---|
| _____ | | |
| _____ | | |
| _____ | | |

**DAILY CALORIES BURNED:** _____

---

### CALORIE CALCULATOR

| _____ | − | _____ | = | _____ | − | _____ | = | _____ |
|---|---|---|---|---|---|---|---|---|
| TOTAL CALORIE INTAKE | | TOTAL CALORIES BURNED | | NET CALORIES | | BMR (Basal Metabolic Rate) | | DAILY NET CALORIE GAIN OR LOSS |

**Energy Level:**
👎 1 2 3 4 5 6 👍

**Muscle Group Worked:**
☐ arms ☐ chest ☐ back ☐ core ☐ thighs ☐ calves

**Diet & Workout Notes:**

_____

_____

_____

_____

# Day 5

DATE:_____    WEIGHT:_____

| BREAKFAST | Qty. | Calories | Fat | Carbs | Other |
|-----------|------|----------|-----|-------|-------|
| _____ | ___ | | | | |
| _____ | ___ | | | | |
| _____ | ___ | | | | |
| _____ | ___ | | | | |
| _____ | ___ | | | | |

| SNACK | Qty. | Calories | Fat | Carbs | Other |
|-------|------|----------|-----|-------|-------|
| _____ | ___ | | | | |
| _____ | ___ | | | | |

| LUNCH | Qty. | Calories | Fat | Carbs | Other |
|-------|------|----------|-----|-------|-------|
| _____ | ___ | | | | |
| _____ | ___ | | | | |
| _____ | ___ | | | | |
| _____ | ___ | | | | |
| _____ | ___ | | | | |

| SNACK | Qty. | Calories | Fat | Carbs | Other |
|-------|------|----------|-----|-------|-------|
| _____ | ___ | | | | |
| _____ | ___ | | | | |

| DINNER | Qty. | Calories | Fat | Carbs | Other |
|--------|------|----------|-----|-------|-------|
| _____ | ___ | | | | |
| _____ | ___ | | | | |
| _____ | ___ | | | | |
| _____ | ___ | | | | |
| _____ | ___ | | | | |

**DAILY INTAKE TOTALS:**

☑ **Water Intake**
# of 8 oz. glasses

**Daily # of Servings**

fruits          meats & beans

veggies         milk & dairy

grains          oils & sweets

**Vitamins & Supplements:**

_____

_____

_____

# FITNESS JOURNAL

DAILY GOAL: _____ GOAL MET: ☐

### 🏃 CARDIOVASCULAR EXERCISE

| | Duration | Distance | Pace | Cal. Burned |
|---|---|---|---|---|
| _____ | | | | |
| _____ | | | | |
| _____ | | | | |
| _____ | | | | |

### 🏋 STRENGTH TRAINING

| | Weight | Reps. | Sets | Cal. Burned |
|---|---|---|---|---|
| _____ | | | | |
| _____ | | | | |
| _____ | | | | |
| _____ | | | | |
| _____ | | | | |
| _____ | | | | |
| _____ | | | | |

### 🤸 FLEXIBILITY, RELAXATION, MEDITATION

| | Duration | Cal. Burned |
|---|---|---|
| _____ | | |
| _____ | | |
| _____ | | |

**DAILY CALORIES BURNED:** _____

---

## CALORIE CALCULATOR

| | | | | |
|---|---|---|---|---|
| _____ − | _____ = | _____ − | _____ = | _____ |
| TOTAL CALORIE INTAKE | TOTAL CALORIES BURNED | NET CALORIES | BMR (Basal Metabolic Rate) | DAILY NET CALORIE GAIN OR LOSS |

---

**Energy Level:**
👎 1 2 3 4 5 6 👍

**Muscle Group Worked:**
☐ arms ☐ chest ☐ back ☐ core ☐ thighs ☐ calves

**Diet & Workout Notes:**

_____
_____
_____
_____

# Day 6

DATE: _____          WEIGHT: _____

| BREAKFAST | Qty. | Calories | Fat | Carbs | Other |
|-----------|------|----------|-----|-------|-------|
| _____ | _____ | | | | |
| _____ | _____ | | | | |
| _____ | _____ | | | | |
| _____ | _____ | | | | |
| _____ | _____ | | | | |

| SNACK | Qty. | Calories | Fat | Carbs | Other |
|-------|------|----------|-----|-------|-------|
| _____ | _____ | | | | |
| _____ | _____ | | | | |

| LUNCH | Qty. | Calories | Fat | Carbs | Other |
|-------|------|----------|-----|-------|-------|
| _____ | _____ | | | | |
| _____ | _____ | | | | |
| _____ | _____ | | | | |
| _____ | _____ | | | | |
| _____ | _____ | | | | |

| SNACK | Qty. | Calories | Fat | Carbs | Other |
|-------|------|----------|-----|-------|-------|
| _____ | _____ | | | | |
| _____ | _____ | | | | |

| DINNER | Qty. | Calories | Fat | Carbs | Other |
|--------|------|----------|-----|-------|-------|
| _____ | _____ | | | | |
| _____ | _____ | | | | |
| _____ | _____ | | | | |
| _____ | _____ | | | | |

**DAILY INTAKE TOTALS:**

☑ **Water Intake**
# of 8 oz. glasses

☐ ☐ ☐
☐ ☐ ☐
☐ ☐ ☐

**Daily # of Servings**

☐ fruits          ☐ meats & beans
☐ veggies        ☐ milk & dairy
☐ grains          ☐ oils & sweets

**Vitamins & Supplements:**

_____

_____

_____

# FITNESS JOURNAL

DAILY GOAL: _____     GOAL MET: ☐

### CARDIOVASCULAR EXERCISE

| | Duration | Distance | Pace | Cal. Burned |
|---|---|---|---|---|
| _____ | | | | |
| _____ | | | | |
| _____ | | | | |
| _____ | | | | |

### STRENGTH TRAINING

| | Weight | Reps. | Sets | Cal. Burned |
|---|---|---|---|---|
| _____ | | | | |
| _____ | | | | |
| _____ | | | | |
| _____ | | | | |
| _____ | | | | |
| _____ | | | | |
| _____ | | | | |
| _____ | | | | |

### FLEXIBILITY, RELAXATION, MEDITATION

| | Duration | Cal. Burned |
|---|---|---|
| _____ | | |
| _____ | | |
| _____ | | |

**DAILY CALORIES BURNED:** _____

---

## CALORIE CALCULATOR

| ____ | − | ____ | = | ____ | − | ____ | = | ____ |
|---|---|---|---|---|---|---|---|---|
| TOTAL CALORIE INTAKE | | TOTAL CALORIES BURNED | | NET CALORIES | | BMR (Basal Metabolic Rate) | | DAILY NET CALORIE GAIN OR LOSS |

---

**Energy Level:**  👎  1  2  3  4  5  6  👍

**Muscle Group Worked:**
☐ arms  ☐ chest  ☐ back  ☐ core  ☐ thighs  ☐ calves

**Diet & Workout Notes:**

_____
_____
_____
_____

# Day 7

DATE: _____          WEIGHT: _____

| 🍎 BREAKFAST | Qty. | Calories | Fat | Carbs | Other |
|---|---|---|---|---|---|
| _____ | _____ | | | | |
| _____ | _____ | | | | |
| _____ | _____ | | | | |
| _____ | _____ | | | | |
| _____ | _____ | | | | |

| ➕ SNACK | Qty. | Calories | Fat | Carbs | Other |
|---|---|---|---|---|---|
| _____ | _____ | | | | |
| _____ | _____ | | | | |

| 🍔 LUNCH | Qty. | Calories | Fat | Carbs | Other |
|---|---|---|---|---|---|
| _____ | _____ | | | | |
| _____ | _____ | | | | |
| _____ | _____ | | | | |
| _____ | _____ | | | | |
| _____ | _____ | | | | |

| 🍇 SNACK | Qty. | Calories | Fat | Carbs | Other |
|---|---|---|---|---|---|
| _____ | _____ | | | | |
| _____ | _____ | | | | |

| 🥄 DINNER | Qty. | Calories | Fat | Carbs | Other |
|---|---|---|---|---|---|
| _____ | _____ | | | | |
| _____ | _____ | | | | |
| _____ | _____ | | | | |
| _____ | _____ | | | | |

**DAILY INTAKE TOTALS:**

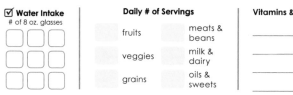

☑ **Water Intake**
# of 8 oz. glasses

**Daily # of Servings**

fruits          meats & beans

veggies          milk & dairy

grains          oils & sweets

**Vitamins & Supplements:**

_____
_____
_____
_____

# FITNESS JOURNAL

DAILY GOAL: _____  GOAL MET: ☐

### CARDIOVASCULAR EXERCISE

| | Duration | Distance | Pace | Cal. Burned |
|---|---|---|---|---|
| _____ | | | | |
| _____ | | | | |
| _____ | | | | |
| _____ | | | | |

### STRENGTH TRAINING

| | Weight | Reps. | Sets | Cal. Burned |
|---|---|---|---|---|
| _____ | | | | |
| _____ | | | | |
| _____ | | | | |
| _____ | | | | |
| _____ | | | | |
| _____ | | | | |
| _____ | | | | |
| _____ | | | | |

### FLEXIBILITY, RELAXATION, MEDITATION

| | Duration | Cal. Burned |
|---|---|---|
| _____ | | |
| _____ | | |
| _____ | | |

**DAILY CALORIES BURNED:**

## CALORIE CALCULATOR

| | | | | |
|---|---|---|---|---|
| ▭ − ▭ | = | ▭ − ▭ | = | ▭ |
| TOTAL CALORIE INTAKE / TOTAL CALORIES BURNED | | NET CALORIES / BMR (Basal Metabolic Rate) | | DAILY NET CALORIE GAIN OR LOSS |

**Energy Level:**
👎 1  2  3  4  5  6  👍

**Muscle Group Worked:**
☐ arms  ☐ chest  ☐ back  ☐ core  ☐ thighs  ☐ calves

**Diet & Workout Notes:**

_____
_____
_____
_____

# Day 8

DATE: _____          WEIGHT: _____

| BREAKFAST | Qty. | Calories | Fat | Carbs | Other |
|---|---|---|---|---|---|
| _____ | ____ | | | | |
| _____ | ____ | | | | |
| _____ | ____ | | | | |
| _____ | ____ | | | | |
| _____ | ____ | | | | |

| SNACK | Qty. | Calories | Fat | Carbs | Other |
|---|---|---|---|---|---|
| _____ | ____ | | | | |
| _____ | ____ | | | | |

| LUNCH | Qty. | Calories | Fat | Carbs | Other |
|---|---|---|---|---|---|
| _____ | ____ | | | | |
| _____ | ____ | | | | |
| _____ | ____ | | | | |
| _____ | ____ | | | | |
| _____ | ____ | | | | |

| SNACK | Qty. | Calories | Fat | Carbs | Other |
|---|---|---|---|---|---|
| _____ | ____ | | | | |
| _____ | ____ | | | | |

| DINNER | Qty. | Calories | Fat | Carbs | Other |
|---|---|---|---|---|---|
| _____ | ____ | | | | |
| _____ | ____ | | | | |
| _____ | ____ | | | | |
| _____ | ____ | | | | |
| _____ | ____ | | | | |

**DAILY INTAKE TOTALS:**

☑ **Water Intake**
# of 8 oz. glasses

☐ ☐ ☐
☐ ☐ ☐
☐ ☐ ☐

**Daily # of Servings**

fruits

veggies

grains

meats & beans

milk & dairy

oils & sweets

**Vitamins & Supplements:**

_____
_____
_____
_____

# FITNESS JOURNAL

DAILY GOAL: _____  GOAL MET: ☐

### CARDIOVASCULAR EXERCISE

| | Duration | Distance | Pace | Cal. Burned |
|---|---|---|---|---|
| _____ | | | | |
| _____ | | | | |
| _____ | | | | |
| _____ | | | | |

### STRENGTH TRAINING

| | Weight | Reps. | Sets | Cal. Burned |
|---|---|---|---|---|
| _____ | | | | |
| _____ | | | | |
| _____ | | | | |
| _____ | | | | |
| _____ | | | | |
| _____ | | | | |
| _____ | | | | |
| _____ | | | | |

### FLEXIBILITY, RELAXATION, MEDITATION

| | Duration | Cal. Burned |
|---|---|---|
| _____ | | |
| _____ | | |
| _____ | | |

**DAILY CALORIES BURNED:**

## CALORIE CALCULATOR

| | − | | = | | − | | = | |
|---|---|---|---|---|---|---|---|---|
| TOTAL CALORIE INTAKE | | TOTAL CALORIES BURNED | | NET CALORIES | | BMR (Basal Metabolic Rate) | | DAILY NET CALORIE GAIN OR LOSS |

**Energy Level:**   1   2   3   4   5   6

**Muscle Group Worked:**  ☐ arms  ☐ chest  ☐ back  ☐ core  ☐ thighs  ☐ calves

**Diet & Workout Notes:**

_____
_____
_____
_____

# Day 9

DATE: _____          WEIGHT: _____

| BREAKFAST | Qty. | Calories | Fat | Carbs | Other |
|---|---|---|---|---|---|
| _____ | _____ | | | | |
| _____ | _____ | | | | |
| _____ | _____ | | | | |
| _____ | _____ | | | | |
| _____ | _____ | | | | |

| SNACK | Qty. | Calories | Fat | Carbs | Other |
|---|---|---|---|---|---|
| _____ | _____ | | | | |
| _____ | _____ | | | | |

| LUNCH | Qty. | Calories | Fat | Carbs | Other |
|---|---|---|---|---|---|
| _____ | _____ | | | | |
| _____ | _____ | | | | |
| _____ | _____ | | | | |
| _____ | _____ | | | | |
| _____ | _____ | | | | |

| SNACK | Qty. | Calories | Fat | Carbs | Other |
|---|---|---|---|---|---|
| _____ | _____ | | | | |
| _____ | _____ | | | | |

| DINNER | Qty. | Calories | Fat | Carbs | Other |
|---|---|---|---|---|---|
| _____ | _____ | | | | |
| _____ | _____ | | | | |
| _____ | _____ | | | | |
| _____ | _____ | | | | |
| _____ | _____ | | | | |

**DAILY INTAKE TOTALS:**

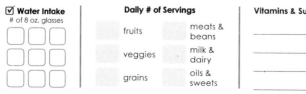

☑ **Water Intake**
# of 8 oz. glasses

**Daily # of Servings**

____ fruits          ____ meats & beans

____ veggies      ____ milk & dairy

____ grains        ____ oils & sweets

**Vitamins & Supplements:**

_____

_____

_____

_____

# FITNESS JOURNAL

DAILY GOAL: _____  GOAL MET: ☐

### 🏃 CARDIOVASCULAR EXERCISE

| | Duration | Distance | Pace | Cal. Burned |
|---|---|---|---|---|
| _____ | | | | |
| _____ | | | | |
| _____ | | | | |
| _____ | | | | |

### 🏋 STRENGTH TRAINING

| | Weight | Reps. | Sets | Cal. Burned |
|---|---|---|---|---|
| _____ | | | | |
| _____ | | | | |
| _____ | | | | |
| _____ | | | | |
| _____ | | | | |
| _____ | | | | |
| _____ | | | | |

### 🧘 FLEXIBILITY, RELAXATION, MEDITATION

| | Duration | Cal. Burned |
|---|---|---|
| _____ | | |
| _____ | | |
| _____ | | |

**DAILY CALORIES BURNED:** _____

---

### CALORIE CALCULATOR

| | | | | | | | |
|---|---|---|---|---|---|---|---|
| _____ | − | _____ | = | _____ | − | _____ | = | _____ |
| TOTAL CALORIE INTAKE | | TOTAL CALORIES BURNED | | NET CALORIES | | BMR (Basal Metabolic Rate) | | DAILY NET CALORIE GAIN OR LOSS |

---

**Energy Level:**  👎 1  2  3  4  5  6  👍

**Muscle Group Worked:** ☐ arms ☐ chest ☐ back ☐ core ☐ thighs ☐ calves

**Diet & Workout Notes:**

_____

_____

_____

_____

# Day 10

DATE: _____          WEIGHT: _____

| BREAKFAST | Qty. | Calories | Fat | Carbs | Other |
|-----------|------|----------|-----|-------|-------|
| | | | | | |
| | | | | | |
| | | | | | |
| | | | | | |
| | | | | | |

| SNACK | Qty. | Calories | Fat | Carbs | Other |
|-------|------|----------|-----|-------|-------|
| | | | | | |
| | | | | | |

| LUNCH | Qty. | Calories | Fat | Carbs | Other |
|-------|------|----------|-----|-------|-------|
| | | | | | |
| | | | | | |
| | | | | | |
| | | | | | |
| | | | | | |

| SNACK | Qty. | Calories | Fat | Carbs | Other |
|-------|------|----------|-----|-------|-------|
| | | | | | |
| | | | | | |

| DINNER | Qty. | Calories | Fat | Carbs | Other |
|--------|------|----------|-----|-------|-------|
| | | | | | |
| | | | | | |
| | | | | | |
| | | | | | |
| | | | | | |

**DAILY INTAKE TOTALS:**

☑ **Water Intake**
# of 8 oz. glasses

**Daily # of Servings**

fruits          meats & beans

veggies         milk & dairy

grains          oils & sweets

**Vitamins & Supplements:**

_____

_____

_____

_____

# FITNESS JOURNAL

DAILY GOAL: _____ GOAL MET: ☐

### 🏃 CARDIOVASCULAR EXERCISE

| | Duration | Distance | Pace | Cal. Burned |
|---|---|---|---|---|
| _____ | | | | |
| _____ | | | | |
| _____ | | | | |
| _____ | | | | |

### 🏋 STRENGTH TRAINING

| | Weight | Reps. | Sets | Cal. Burned |
|---|---|---|---|---|
| _____ | | | | |
| _____ | | | | |
| _____ | | | | |
| _____ | | | | |
| _____ | | | | |
| _____ | | | | |
| _____ | | | | |
| _____ | | | | |

### 🧘 FLEXIBILITY, RELAXATION, MEDITATION

| | Duration | Cal. Burned |
|---|---|---|
| _____ | | |
| _____ | | |
| _____ | | |

**DAILY CALORIES BURNED:** _____

---

## CALORIE CALCULATOR

| _____ | − | _____ | = | _____ | − | _____ | = | _____ |
|---|---|---|---|---|---|---|---|---|
| TOTAL CALORIE INTAKE | | TOTAL CALORIES BURNED | | NET CALORIES | | BMR (Basal Metabolic Rate) | | DAILY NET CALORIE GAIN OR LOSS |

**Energy Level:**
👎 1  2  3  4  5  6 👍

**Muscle Group Worked:**
☐ arms ☐ chest ☐ back ☐ core ☐ thighs ☐ calves

**Diet & Workout Notes:**

_____
_____
_____
_____

# Day 11

DATE: _____          WEIGHT: _____

| BREAKFAST | Qty. | Calories | Fat | Carbs | Other |
|---|---|---|---|---|---|
| _____ | ____ | | | | |
| _____ | ____ | | | | |
| _____ | ____ | | | | |
| _____ | ____ | | | | |
| _____ | ____ | | | | |

| SNACK | Qty. | Calories | Fat | Carbs | Other |
|---|---|---|---|---|---|
| _____ | ____ | | | | |
| _____ | ____ | | | | |

| LUNCH | Qty. | Calories | Fat | Carbs | Other |
|---|---|---|---|---|---|
| _____ | ____ | | | | |
| _____ | ____ | | | | |
| _____ | ____ | | | | |
| _____ | ____ | | | | |
| _____ | ____ | | | | |

| SNACK | Qty. | Calories | Fat | Carbs | Other |
|---|---|---|---|---|---|
| _____ | ____ | | | | |
| _____ | ____ | | | | |

| DINNER | Qty. | Calories | Fat | Carbs | Other |
|---|---|---|---|---|---|
| _____ | ____ | | | | |
| _____ | ____ | | | | |
| _____ | ____ | | | | |
| _____ | ____ | | | | |
| _____ | ____ | | | | |

**DAILY INTAKE TOTALS:**

☑ **Water Intake**
# of 8 oz. glasses

☐ ☐ ☐
☐ ☐ ☐
☐ ☐ ☐

**Daily # of Servings**

fruits

veggies

grains

meats & beans

milk & dairy

oils & sweets

**Vitamins & Supplements:**

_____
_____
_____
_____

# FITNESS JOURNAL

DAILY GOAL: _____  GOAL MET: ☐

### CARDIOVASCULAR EXERCISE

| | Duration | Distance | Pace | Cal. Burned |
|---|---|---|---|---|
| | | | | |
| | | | | |
| | | | | |
| | | | | |

### STRENGTH TRAINING

| | Weight | Reps. | Sets | Cal. Burned |
|---|---|---|---|---|
| | | | | |
| | | | | |
| | | | | |
| | | | | |
| | | | | |
| | | | | |
| | | | | |
| | | | | |

### FLEXIBILITY, RELAXATION, MEDITATION

| | Duration | Cal. Burned |
|---|---|---|
| | | |
| | | |
| | | |

**DAILY CALORIES BURNED:**

## CALORIE CALCULATOR

|   | − |   | = |   | − |   | = |   |
|---|---|---|---|---|---|---|---|---|
| TOTAL CALORIE INTAKE | | TOTAL CALORIES BURNED | | NET CALORIES | | BMR (Basal Metabolic Rate) | | DAILY NET CALORIE GAIN OR LOSS |

**Energy Level:**
1   2   3   4   5   6

**Muscle Group Worked:**
☐ arms  ☐ chest  ☐ back  ☐ core  ☐ thighs  ☐ calves

**Diet & Workout Notes:**

_____
_____
_____
_____

# Day 12

DATE: _____    WEIGHT: _____

| BREAKFAST | Qty. | Calories | Fat | Carbs | Other |
|---|---|---|---|---|---|
| _____ | ____ | | | | |
| _____ | ____ | | | | |
| _____ | ____ | | | | |
| _____ | ____ | | | | |
| _____ | ____ | | | | |

| SNACK | Qty. | Calories | Fat | Carbs | Other |
|---|---|---|---|---|---|
| _____ | ____ | | | | |
| _____ | ____ | | | | |

| LUNCH | Qty. | Calories | Fat | Carbs | Other |
|---|---|---|---|---|---|
| _____ | ____ | | | | |
| _____ | ____ | | | | |
| _____ | ____ | | | | |
| _____ | ____ | | | | |
| _____ | ____ | | | | |

| SNACK | Qty. | Calories | Fat | Carbs | Other |
|---|---|---|---|---|---|
| _____ | ____ | | | | |
| _____ | ____ | | | | |

| DINNER | Qty. | Calories | Fat | Carbs | Other |
|---|---|---|---|---|---|
| _____ | ____ | | | | |
| _____ | ____ | | | | |
| _____ | ____ | | | | |
| _____ | ____ | | | | |
| _____ | ____ | | | | |

**DAILY INTAKE TOTALS:**

☑ **Water Intake**
# of 8 oz. glasses

**Daily # of Servings**

- fruits
- veggies
- grains
- meats & beans
- milk & dairy
- oils & sweets

**Vitamins & Supplements:**

_____
_____
_____
_____

# FITNESS JOURNAL

**DAILY GOAL:** _____  **GOAL MET:** ☐

### CARDIOVASCULAR EXERCISE

| | Duration | Distance | Pace | Cal. Burned |
|---|---|---|---|---|
| _____ | | | | |
| _____ | | | | |
| _____ | | | | |
| _____ | | | | |

### STRENGTH TRAINING

| | Weight | Reps. | Sets | Cal. Burned |
|---|---|---|---|---|
| _____ | | | | |
| _____ | | | | |
| _____ | | | | |
| _____ | | | | |
| _____ | | | | |
| _____ | | | | |
| _____ | | | | |

### FLEXIBILITY, RELAXATION, MEDITATION

| | Duration | Cal. Burned |
|---|---|---|
| _____ | | |
| _____ | | |
| _____ | | |

**DAILY CALORIES BURNED:** _____

## CALORIE CALCULATOR

| TOTAL CALORIE INTAKE | − | TOTAL CALORIES BURNED | = | NET CALORIES | − | BMR (Basal Metabolic Rate) | = | DAILY NET CALORIE GAIN OR LOSS |
|---|---|---|---|---|---|---|---|---|

**Energy Level:**  👎  1   2   3   4   5   6  👍

**Muscle Group Worked:**  ☐ arms  ☐ chest  ☐ back  ☐ core  ☐ thighs  ☐ calves

**Diet & Workout Notes:**

_____
_____
_____
_____

# Day 13

**DATE:** _____     **WEIGHT:** _____

| BREAKFAST | Qty. | Calories | Fat | Carbs | Other |
|-----------|------|----------|-----|-------|-------|
| _____ | _____ | | | | |
| _____ | _____ | | | | |
| _____ | _____ | | | | |
| _____ | _____ | | | | |
| _____ | _____ | | | | |

| SNACK | Qty. | Calories | Fat | Carbs | Other |
|-------|------|----------|-----|-------|-------|
| _____ | _____ | | | | |
| _____ | _____ | | | | |

| LUNCH | Qty. | Calories | Fat | Carbs | Other |
|-------|------|----------|-----|-------|-------|
| _____ | _____ | | | | |
| _____ | _____ | | | | |
| _____ | _____ | | | | |
| _____ | _____ | | | | |
| _____ | _____ | | | | |

| SNACK | Qty. | Calories | Fat | Carbs | Other |
|-------|------|----------|-----|-------|-------|
| _____ | _____ | | | | |
| _____ | _____ | | | | |

| DINNER | Qty. | Calories | Fat | Carbs | Other |
|--------|------|----------|-----|-------|-------|
| _____ | _____ | | | | |
| _____ | _____ | | | | |
| _____ | _____ | | | | |
| _____ | _____ | | | | |
| _____ | _____ | | | | |

**DAILY INTAKE TOTALS:**

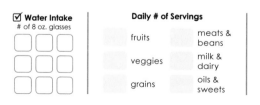

☑ **Water Intake**
# of 8 oz. glasses

**Daily # of Servings**

fruits

veggies

grains

meats & beans

milk & dairy

oils & sweets

**Vitamins & Supplements:**

_____

_____

_____

_____

# FITNESS JOURNAL

DAILY GOAL: _____ GOAL MET: ☐

### 🏃 CARDIOVASCULAR EXERCISE

| | Duration | Distance | Pace | Cal. Burned |
|---|---|---|---|---|
| _____ | | | | |
| _____ | | | | |
| _____ | | | | |
| _____ | | | | |

### 🏋 STRENGTH TRAINING

| | Weight | Reps. | Sets | Cal. Burned |
|---|---|---|---|---|
| _____ | | | | |
| _____ | | | | |
| _____ | | | | |
| _____ | | | | |
| _____ | | | | |
| _____ | | | | |
| _____ | | | | |
| _____ | | | | |

### 🧘 FLEXIBILITY, RELAXATION, MEDITATION

| | Duration | Cal. Burned |
|---|---|---|
| _____ | | |
| _____ | | |
| _____ | | |

**DAILY CALORIES BURNED:**

---

### CALORIE CALCULATOR

| | | | | |
|---|---|---|---|---|
| ▭ − | ▭ = | ▭ − | ▭ = | ▭ |
| TOTAL CALORIE INTAKE | TOTAL CALORIES BURNED | NET CALORIES | BMR (Basal Metabolic Rate) | DAILY NET CALORIE GAIN OR LOSS |

---

**Energy Level:**

👎 1  2  3  4  5  6 👍

**Muscle Group Worked:**

☐ arms  ☐ chest  ☐ back  ☐ core  ☐ thighs  ☐ calves

**Diet & Workout Notes:**

_____

_____

_____

_____

# Day 14

DATE: _____          WEIGHT: _____

| 🍎 BREAKFAST | Qty. | Calories | Fat | Carbs | Other |
|---|---|---|---|---|---|
| _____ | _____ | | | | |
| _____ | _____ | | | | |
| _____ | _____ | | | | |
| _____ | _____ | | | | |
| _____ | _____ | | | | |

| 🍴 SNACK | Qty. | Calories | Fat | Carbs | Other |
|---|---|---|---|---|---|
| _____ | _____ | | | | |
| _____ | _____ | | | | |

| 🍞 LUNCH | Qty. | Calories | Fat | Carbs | Other |
|---|---|---|---|---|---|
| _____ | _____ | | | | |
| _____ | _____ | | | | |
| _____ | _____ | | | | |
| _____ | _____ | | | | |
| _____ | _____ | | | | |

| 🍇 SNACK | Qty. | Calories | Fat | Carbs | Other |
|---|---|---|---|---|---|
| _____ | _____ | | | | |
| _____ | _____ | | | | |

| 🥄 DINNER | Qty. | Calories | Fat | Carbs | Other |
|---|---|---|---|---|---|
| _____ | _____ | | | | |
| _____ | _____ | | | | |
| _____ | _____ | | | | |
| _____ | _____ | | | | |
| _____ | _____ | | | | |

**DAILY INTAKE TOTALS:**

☑ **Water Intake**
# of 8 oz. glasses

☐ ☐ ☐
☐ ☐ ☐
☐ ☐ ☐

**Daily # of Servings**

| | fruits | | meats & beans |
| | veggies | | milk & dairy |
| | grains | | oils & sweets |

**Vitamins & Supplements:**

_____
_____
_____
_____

# FITNESS JOURNAL

**DAILY GOAL:** _____ **GOAL MET:** ☐

### CARDIOVASCULAR EXERCISE

| | Duration | Distance | Pace | Cal. Burned |
|---|---|---|---|---|
| _____ | | | | |
| _____ | | | | |
| _____ | | | | |
| _____ | | | | |

### STRENGTH TRAINING

| | Weight | Reps. | Sets | Cal. Burned |
|---|---|---|---|---|
| _____ | | | | |
| _____ | | | | |
| _____ | | | | |
| _____ | | | | |
| _____ | | | | |
| _____ | | | | |
| _____ | | | | |
| _____ | | | | |

### FLEXIBILITY, RELAXATION, MEDITATION

| | Duration | Cal. Burned |
|---|---|---|
| _____ | | |
| _____ | | |
| _____ | | |

**DAILY CALORIES BURNED:** _____

---

### CALORIE CALCULATOR

| _____ | − | _____ | = | _____ | − | _____ | = | _____ |
|---|---|---|---|---|---|---|---|---|
| TOTAL CALORIE INTAKE | | TOTAL CALORIES BURNED | | NET CALORIES | | BMR (Basal Metabolic Rate) | | DAILY NET CALORIE GAIN OR LOSS |

**Energy Level:** 👎 1 2 3 4 5 6 👍

**Muscle Group Worked:** ☐ arms ☐ chest ☐ back ☐ core ☐ thighs ☐ calves

**Diet & Workout Notes:**

_____

_____

_____

_____

# Day 15

DATE: _____     WEIGHT: _____

### BREAKFAST

| | Qty. | Calories | Fat | Carbs | Other |
|---|---|---|---|---|---|
| _____ | _____ | | | | |
| _____ | _____ | | | | |
| _____ | _____ | | | | |
| _____ | _____ | | | | |
| _____ | _____ | | | | |

### SNACK

| | Qty. | Calories | Fat | Carbs | Other |
|---|---|---|---|---|---|
| _____ | _____ | | | | |
| _____ | _____ | | | | |

### LUNCH

| | Qty. | Calories | Fat | Carbs | Other |
|---|---|---|---|---|---|
| _____ | _____ | | | | |
| _____ | _____ | | | | |
| _____ | _____ | | | | |
| _____ | _____ | | | | |
| _____ | _____ | | | | |

### SNACK

| | Qty. | Calories | Fat | Carbs | Other |
|---|---|---|---|---|---|
| _____ | _____ | | | | |
| _____ | _____ | | | | |

### DINNER

| | Qty. | Calories | Fat | Carbs | Other |
|---|---|---|---|---|---|
| _____ | _____ | | | | |
| _____ | _____ | | | | |
| _____ | _____ | | | | |
| _____ | _____ | | | | |
| _____ | _____ | | | | |

**DAILY INTAKE TOTALS:**

☑ **Water Intake**
# of 8 oz. glasses

**Daily # of Servings**

- fruits
- veggies
- grains
- meats & beans
- milk & dairy
- oils & sweets

**Vitamins & Supplements:**
_____
_____
_____
_____

# FITNESS JOURNAL

**DAILY GOAL:** _____  **GOAL MET:** ☐

### 🏃 CARDIOVASCULAR EXERCISE

| | Duration | Distance | Pace | Cal. Burned |
|---|---|---|---|---|
| _____ | | | | |
| _____ | | | | |
| _____ | | | | |
| _____ | | | | |

### 🏋 STRENGTH TRAINING

| | Weight | Reps. | Sets | Cal. Burned |
|---|---|---|---|---|
| _____ | | | | |
| _____ | | | | |
| _____ | | | | |
| _____ | | | | |
| _____ | | | | |
| _____ | | | | |
| _____ | | | | |
| _____ | | | | |

### 🧘 FLEXIBILITY, RELAXATION, MEDITATION

| | Duration | Cal. Burned |
|---|---|---|
| _____ | | |
| _____ | | |
| _____ | | |

**DAILY CALORIES BURNED:** _____

---

### CALORIE CALCULATOR

| _____ | − | _____ | = | _____ | − | _____ | = | _____ |
|---|---|---|---|---|---|---|---|---|
| TOTAL CALORIE INTAKE | | TOTAL CALORIES BURNED | | NET CALORIES | | BMR (Basal Metabolic Rate) | | DAILY NET CALORIE GAIN OR LOSS |

**Energy Level:** 👎 1  2  3  4  5  6 👍

**Muscle Group Worked:** ☐ arms ☐ chest ☐ back ☐ core ☐ thighs ☐ calves

**Diet & Workout Notes:**

_____

_____

_____

_____

# Day 16

DATE: _____          WEIGHT: _____

| 🍎 BREAKFAST | Qty. | Calories | Fat | Carbs | Other |
|---|---|---|---|---|---|
| _____ | ____ | | | | |
| _____ | ____ | | | | |
| _____ | ____ | | | | |
| _____ | ____ | | | | |
| _____ | ____ | | | | |

| 🥛 SNACK | Qty. | Calories | Fat | Carbs | Other |
|---|---|---|---|---|---|
| _____ | ____ | | | | |
| _____ | ____ | | | | |

| 🍞 LUNCH | Qty. | Calories | Fat | Carbs | Other |
|---|---|---|---|---|---|
| _____ | ____ | | | | |
| _____ | ____ | | | | |
| _____ | ____ | | | | |
| _____ | ____ | | | | |
| _____ | ____ | | | | |

| 🍇 SNACK | Qty. | Calories | Fat | Carbs | Other |
|---|---|---|---|---|---|
| _____ | ____ | | | | |
| _____ | ____ | | | | |

| 🥄 DINNER | Qty. | Calories | Fat | Carbs | Other |
|---|---|---|---|---|---|
| _____ | ____ | | | | |
| _____ | ____ | | | | |
| _____ | ____ | | | | |
| _____ | ____ | | | | |
| _____ | ____ | | | | |

**DAILY INTAKE TOTALS:**

☑ **Water Intake**
# of 8 oz. glasses

☐ ☐ ☐
☐ ☐ ☐
☐ ☐ ☐

**Daily # of Servings**

fruits          meats & beans

veggies         milk & dairy

grains          oils & sweets

**Vitamins & Supplements:**

_____
_____
_____
_____

# FITNESS JOURNAL

DAILY GOAL: _____ GOAL MET: ☐

### CARDIOVASCULAR EXERCISE

| | Duration | Distance | Pace | Cal. Burned |
|---|---|---|---|---|
| | | | | |
| | | | | |
| | | | | |
| | | | | |

### STRENGTH TRAINING

| | Weight | Reps. | Sets | Cal. Burned |
|---|---|---|---|---|
| | | | | |
| | | | | |
| | | | | |
| | | | | |
| | | | | |
| | | | | |
| | | | | |
| | | | | |

### FLEXIBILITY, RELAXATION, MEDITATION

| | Duration | Cal. Burned |
|---|---|---|
| | | |
| | | |
| | | |

**DAILY CALORIES BURNED:** _____

### CALORIE CALCULATOR

| | | | | | | | | |
|---|---|---|---|---|---|---|---|---|
| TOTAL CALORIE INTAKE | − | TOTAL CALORIES BURNED | = | NET CALORIES | − | BMR (Basal Metabolic Rate) | = | DAILY NET CALORIE GAIN OR LOSS |

**Energy Level:** 👎 1 2 3 4 5 6 👍

**Muscle Group Worked:** ☐ arms ☐ chest ☐ back ☐ core ☐ thighs ☐ calves

**Diet & Workout Notes:**

_____
_____
_____
_____

# Day 17

DATE: _____     WEIGHT: _____

| BREAKFAST | Qty. | Calories | Fat | Carbs | Other |
|-----------|------|----------|-----|-------|-------|
| _____ | _____ | | | | |
| _____ | _____ | | | | |
| _____ | _____ | | | | |
| _____ | _____ | | | | |
| _____ | _____ | | | | |

| SNACK | Qty. | Calories | Fat | Carbs | Other |
|-------|------|----------|-----|-------|-------|
| _____ | _____ | | | | |
| _____ | _____ | | | | |

| LUNCH | Qty. | Calories | Fat | Carbs | Other |
|-------|------|----------|-----|-------|-------|
| _____ | _____ | | | | |
| _____ | _____ | | | | |
| _____ | _____ | | | | |
| _____ | _____ | | | | |
| _____ | _____ | | | | |

| SNACK | Qty. | Calories | Fat | Carbs | Other |
|-------|------|----------|-----|-------|-------|
| _____ | _____ | | | | |
| _____ | _____ | | | | |

| DINNER | Qty. | Calories | Fat | Carbs | Other |
|--------|------|----------|-----|-------|-------|
| _____ | _____ | | | | |
| _____ | _____ | | | | |
| _____ | _____ | | | | |
| _____ | _____ | | | | |
| _____ | _____ | | | | |

**DAILY INTAKE TOTALS:**

☑ **Water Intake**
# of 8 oz. glasses

☐ ☐ ☐
☐ ☐ ☐
☐ ☐ ☐

**Daily # of Servings**

☐ fruits          ☐ meats & beans

☐ veggies      ☐ milk & dairy

☐ grains        ☐ oils & sweets

**Vitamins & Supplements:**

_____

_____

_____

_____

# FITNESS JOURNAL

DAILY GOAL: _____ GOAL MET: ☐

### CARDIOVASCULAR EXERCISE

| | Duration | Distance | Pace | Cal. Burned |
|---|---|---|---|---|
| | | | | |
| | | | | |
| | | | | |
| | | | | |

### STRENGTH TRAINING

| | Weight | Reps. | Sets | Cal. Burned |
|---|---|---|---|---|
| | | | | |
| | | | | |
| | | | | |
| | | | | |
| | | | | |
| | | | | |
| | | | | |
| | | | | |

### FLEXIBILITY, RELAXATION, MEDITATION

| | Duration | Cal. Burned |
|---|---|---|
| | | |
| | | |
| | | |

**DAILY CALORIES BURNED:**

---

**CALORIE CALCULATOR**

[ ] − [ ] = [ ] − [ ] = [ ]

| TOTAL CALORIE INTAKE | TOTAL CALORIES BURNED | NET CALORIES | BMR (Basal Metabolic Rate) | DAILY NET CALORIE GAIN OR LOSS |

---

**Energy Level:**
👎 1  2  3  4  5  6 👍

**Muscle Group Worked:**
☐ arms ☐ chest ☐ back ☐ core ☐ thighs ☐ calves

**Diet & Workout Notes:**

_____
_____
_____
_____

# Day 18

DATE: _____          WEIGHT: _____

### 🍎 BREAKFAST

| | Qty. | Calories | Fat | Carbs | Other |
|---|---|---|---|---|---|
| _____ | _____ | | | | |
| _____ | _____ | | | | |
| _____ | _____ | | | | |
| _____ | _____ | | | | |
| _____ | _____ | | | | |

### 🥛 SNACK

| | Qty. | Calories | Fat | Carbs | Other |
|---|---|---|---|---|---|
| _____ | _____ | | | | |
| _____ | _____ | | | | |

### 🍞 LUNCH

| | Qty. | Calories | Fat | Carbs | Other |
|---|---|---|---|---|---|
| _____ | _____ | | | | |
| _____ | _____ | | | | |
| _____ | _____ | | | | |
| _____ | _____ | | | | |
| _____ | _____ | | | | |

### 🍇 SNACK

| | Qty. | Calories | Fat | Carbs | Other |
|---|---|---|---|---|---|
| _____ | _____ | | | | |
| _____ | _____ | | | | |

### 🍳 DINNER

| | Qty. | Calories | Fat | Carbs | Other |
|---|---|---|---|---|---|
| _____ | _____ | | | | |
| _____ | _____ | | | | |
| _____ | _____ | | | | |
| _____ | _____ | | | | |

**DAILY INTAKE TOTALS:**

☑ **Water Intake**
# of 8 oz. glasses

**Daily # of Servings**

| | |
|---|---|
| fruits | meats & beans |
| veggies | milk & dairy |
| grains | oils & sweets |

**Vitamins & Supplements:**

_____

_____

_____

_____

# FITNESS JOURNAL

DAILY GOAL: _____ GOAL MET: ☐

### CARDIOVASCULAR EXERCISE

| | Duration | Distance | Pace | Cal. Burned |
|---|---|---|---|---|
| _____ | | | | |
| _____ | | | | |
| _____ | | | | |
| _____ | | | | |

### STRENGTH TRAINING

| | Weight | Reps. | Sets | Cal. Burned |
|---|---|---|---|---|
| _____ | | | | |
| _____ | | | | |
| _____ | | | | |
| _____ | | | | |
| _____ | | | | |
| _____ | | | | |
| _____ | | | | |
| _____ | | | | |

### FLEXIBILITY, RELAXATION, MEDITATION

| | Duration | Cal. Burned |
|---|---|---|
| _____ | | |
| _____ | | |
| _____ | | |

**DAILY CALORIES BURNED:** _____

---

### CALORIE CALCULATOR

| _____ | − | _____ | = | _____ | − | _____ | = | _____ |
|---|---|---|---|---|---|---|---|---|
| TOTAL CALORIE INTAKE | | TOTAL CALORIES BURNED | | NET CALORIES | | BMR (Basal Metabolic Rate) | | DAILY NET CALORIE GAIN OR LOSS |

**Energy Level:**
👎 1  2  3  4  5  6 👍

**Muscle Group Worked:**
☐ arms  ☐ chest  ☐ back  ☐ core  ☐ thighs  ☐ calves

**Diet & Workout Notes:**

_____

_____

_____

_____

# Day 19

DATE:_____     WEIGHT:_____

| BREAKFAST | Qty. | Calories | Fat | Carbs | Other |
|---|---|---|---|---|---|
| | | | | | |
| | | | | | |
| | | | | | |
| | | | | | |
| | | | | | |

| SNACK | Qty. | Calories | Fat | Carbs | Other |
|---|---|---|---|---|---|
| | | | | | |
| | | | | | |

| LUNCH | Qty. | Calories | Fat | Carbs | Other |
|---|---|---|---|---|---|
| | | | | | |
| | | | | | |
| | | | | | |
| | | | | | |
| | | | | | |

| SNACK | Qty. | Calories | Fat | Carbs | Other |
|---|---|---|---|---|---|
| | | | | | |
| | | | | | |

| DINNER | Qty. | Calories | Fat | Carbs | Other |
|---|---|---|---|---|---|
| | | | | | |
| | | | | | |
| | | | | | |
| | | | | | |

**DAILY INTAKE TOTALS:**

☑ **Water Intake**
# of 8 oz. glasses

**Daily # of Servings**

fruits    meats & beans

veggies    milk & dairy

grains    oils & sweets

**Vitamins & Supplements:**
_____
_____
_____
_____

# FITNESS JOURNAL

DAILY GOAL: _____ GOAL MET: ☐

### 🏃 CARDIOVASCULAR EXERCISE

| | Duration | Distance | Pace | Cal. Burned |
|---|---|---|---|---|
| | | | | |
| | | | | |
| | | | | |
| | | | | |

### 🏋 STRENGTH TRAINING

| | Weight | Reps. | Sets | Cal. Burned |
|---|---|---|---|---|
| | | | | |
| | | | | |
| | | | | |
| | | | | |
| | | | | |
| | | | | |
| | | | | |
| | | | | |

### 方 FLEXIBILITY, RELAXATION, MEDITATION

| | Duration | Cal. Burned |
|---|---|---|
| | | |
| | | |
| | | |

**DAILY CALORIES BURNED:** _____

---

## CALORIE CALCULATOR

| _____ − _____ = _____ − _____ = _____ |
|---|

| TOTAL CALORIE INTAKE | TOTAL CALORIES BURNED | NET CALORIES | BMR (Basal Metabolic Rate) | DAILY NET CALORIE GAIN OR LOSS |

---

**Energy Level:**
👎 1 2 3 4 5 6 👍

**Muscle Group Worked:**
☐ arms ☐ chest ☐ back ☐ core ☐ thighs ☐ calves

**Diet & Workout Notes:**

_____

_____

_____

_____

# Day 20

DATE: _____     WEIGHT: _____

| BREAKFAST | Qty. | Calories | Fat | Carbs | Other |
|-----------|------|----------|-----|-------|-------|
| _____ | _____ | | | | |
| _____ | _____ | | | | |
| _____ | _____ | | | | |
| _____ | _____ | | | | |
| _____ | _____ | | | | |

| SNACK | Qty. | Calories | Fat | Carbs | Other |
|-------|------|----------|-----|-------|-------|
| _____ | _____ | | | | |
| _____ | _____ | | | | |

| LUNCH | Qty. | Calories | Fat | Carbs | Other |
|-------|------|----------|-----|-------|-------|
| _____ | _____ | | | | |
| _____ | _____ | | | | |
| _____ | _____ | | | | |
| _____ | _____ | | | | |
| _____ | _____ | | | | |

| SNACK | Qty. | Calories | Fat | Carbs | Other |
|-------|------|----------|-----|-------|-------|
| _____ | _____ | | | | |
| _____ | _____ | | | | |

| DINNER | Qty. | Calories | Fat | Carbs | Other |
|--------|------|----------|-----|-------|-------|
| _____ | _____ | | | | |
| _____ | _____ | | | | |
| _____ | _____ | | | | |
| _____ | _____ | | | | |
| _____ | _____ | | | | |

**DAILY INTAKE TOTALS:**

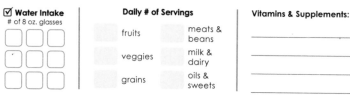

☑ **Water Intake**
# of 8 oz. glasses

**Daily # of Servings**

fruits          meats & beans

veggies       milk & dairy

grains         oils & sweets

**Vitamins & Supplements:**

_____

_____

_____

# FITNESS JOURNAL

DAILY GOAL: _____  GOAL MET: ☐

### 🏃 CARDIOVASCULAR EXERCISE

| | Duration | Distance | Pace | Cal. Burned |
|---|---|---|---|---|
| | | | | |
| | | | | |
| | | | | |
| | | | | |

### 🏋 STRENGTH TRAINING

| | Weight | Reps. | Sets | Cal. Burned |
|---|---|---|---|---|
| | | | | |
| | | | | |
| | | | | |
| | | | | |
| | | | | |
| | | | | |
| | | | | |
| | | | | |

### 方 FLEXIBILITY, RELAXATION, MEDITATION

| | Duration | Cal. Burned |
|---|---|---|
| | | |
| | | |
| | | |

**DAILY CALORIES BURNED:** ____

---

## CALORIE CALCULATOR

| ____ | − | ____ | = | ____ | − | ____ | = | ____ |
|---|---|---|---|---|---|---|---|---|
| TOTAL CALORIE INTAKE | | TOTAL CALORIES BURNED | | NET CALORIES | | BMR (Basal Metabolic Rate) | | DAILY NET CALORIE GAIN OR LOSS |

**Energy Level:**  👎  1  2  3  4  5  6  👍

**Muscle Group Worked:**  ☐ arms  ☐ chest  ☐ back  ☐ core  ☐ thighs  ☐ calves

**Diet & Workout Notes:**

_____

_____

_____

_____

# Day 21

DATE: _____          WEIGHT: _____

| BREAKFAST | Qty. | Calories | Fat | Carbs | Other |
|---|---|---|---|---|---|
| _____ | ____ | | | | |
| _____ | ____ | | | | |
| _____ | ____ | | | | |
| _____ | ____ | | | | |
| _____ | ____ | | | | |

| SNACK | Qty. | Calories | Fat | Carbs | Other |
|---|---|---|---|---|---|
| _____ | ____ | | | | |
| _____ | ____ | | | | |

| LUNCH | Qty. | Calories | Fat | Carbs | Other |
|---|---|---|---|---|---|
| _____ | ____ | | | | |
| _____ | ____ | | | | |
| _____ | ____ | | | | |
| _____ | ____ | | | | |
| _____ | ____ | | | | |

| SNACK | Qty. | Calories | Fat | Carbs | Other |
|---|---|---|---|---|---|
| _____ | ____ | | | | |
| _____ | ____ | | | | |

| DINNER | Qty. | Calories | Fat | Carbs | Other |
|---|---|---|---|---|---|
| _____ | ____ | | | | |
| _____ | ____ | | | | |
| _____ | ____ | | | | |
| _____ | ____ | | | | |

**DAILY INTAKE TOTALS:**

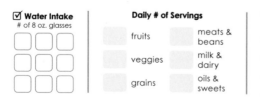

☑ **Water Intake**
# of 8 oz. glasses

**Daily # of Servings**

- _____ fruits
- _____ veggies
- _____ grains
- _____ meats & beans
- _____ milk & dairy
- _____ oils & sweets

**Vitamins & Supplements:**
_____
_____
_____
_____

# FITNESS JOURNAL

DAILY GOAL: _____     GOAL MET: ☐

### CARDIOVASCULAR EXERCISE

| | Duration | Distance | Pace | Cal. Burned |
|---|---|---|---|---|
| _____ | | | | |
| _____ | | | | |
| _____ | | | | |
| _____ | | | | |

### STRENGTH TRAINING

| | Weight | Reps. | Sets | Cal. Burned |
|---|---|---|---|---|
| _____ | | | | |
| _____ | | | | |
| _____ | | | | |
| _____ | | | | |
| _____ | | | | |
| _____ | | | | |
| _____ | | | | |
| _____ | | | | |

### FLEXIBILITY, RELAXATION, MEDITATION

| | Duration | Cal. Burned |
|---|---|---|
| _____ | | |
| _____ | | |
| _____ | | |

**DAILY CALORIES BURNED:** _____

---

## CALORIE CALCULATOR

| _____ | − | _____ | = | _____ | − | _____ | = | _____ |
|---|---|---|---|---|---|---|---|---|
| TOTAL CALORIE INTAKE | | TOTAL CALORIES BURNED | | NET CALORIES | | BMR (Basal Metabolic Rate) | | DAILY NET CALORIE GAIN OR LOSS |

**Energy Level:**   👎  1   2   3   4   5   6  👍

**Muscle Group Worked:** ☐ arms  ☐ chest  ☐ back  ☐ core  ☐ thighs  ☐ calves

**Diet & Workout Notes:**

_____

_____

_____

_____

# Day 22

DATE: _____          WEIGHT: _____

| BREAKFAST | Qty. | Calories | Fat | Carbs | Other |
|-----------|------|----------|-----|-------|-------|
| | | | | | |
| | | | | | |
| | | | | | |
| | | | | | |
| | | | | | |

| SNACK | Qty. | Calories | Fat | Carbs | Other |
|-------|------|----------|-----|-------|-------|
| | | | | | |
| | | | | | |

| LUNCH | Qty. | Calories | Fat | Carbs | Other |
|-------|------|----------|-----|-------|-------|
| | | | | | |
| | | | | | |
| | | | | | |
| | | | | | |
| | | | | | |

| SNACK | Qty. | Calories | Fat | Carbs | Other |
|-------|------|----------|-----|-------|-------|
| | | | | | |
| | | | | | |

| DINNER | Qty. | Calories | Fat | Carbs | Other |
|--------|------|----------|-----|-------|-------|
| | | | | | |
| | | | | | |
| | | | | | |
| | | | | | |
| | | | | | |

**DAILY INTAKE TOTALS:**

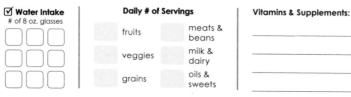

☑ **Water Intake**
# of 8 oz. glasses

**Daily # of Servings**

fruits          meats & beans

veggies          milk & dairy

grains          oils & sweets

**Vitamins & Supplements:**

_____

_____

_____

_____

# FITNESS JOURNAL

**DAILY GOAL:** _____   **GOAL MET:** ☐

### 🏃 CARDIOVASCULAR EXERCISE

| | Duration | Distance | Pace | Cal. Burned |
|---|---|---|---|---|
| _____ | | | | |
| _____ | | | | |
| _____ | | | | |
| _____ | | | | |

### 🏋 STRENGTH TRAINING

| | Weight | Reps. | Sets | Cal. Burned |
|---|---|---|---|---|
| _____ | | | | |
| _____ | | | | |
| _____ | | | | |
| _____ | | | | |
| _____ | | | | |
| _____ | | | | |
| _____ | | | | |
| _____ | | | | |

### 方 FLEXIBILITY, RELAXATION, MEDITATION

| | Duration | Cal. Burned |
|---|---|---|
| _____ | | |
| _____ | | |
| _____ | | |

**DAILY CALORIES BURNED:** [____]

## CALORIE CALCULATOR

| [____] | − | [____] | = | [____] | − | [____] | = | [____] |
|---|---|---|---|---|---|---|---|---|
| TOTAL CALORIE INTAKE | | TOTAL CALORIES BURNED | | NET CALORIES | | BMR (Basal Metabolic Rate) | | DAILY NET CALORIE GAIN OR LOSS |

**Energy Level:**  👎  1  2  3  4  5  6  👍

**Muscle Group Worked:**  ☐ arms  ☐ chest  ☐ back  ☐ core  ☐ thighs  ☐ calves

**Diet & Workout Notes:**

_____

_____

_____

_____

# Day 23

DATE: _____    WEIGHT: _____

| BREAKFAST | Qty. | Calories | Fat | Carbs | Other |
|-----------|------|----------|-----|-------|-------|
| _____ | _____ | | | | |
| _____ | _____ | | | | |
| _____ | _____ | | | | |
| _____ | _____ | | | | |
| _____ | _____ | | | | |

| SNACK | Qty. | Calories | Fat | Carbs | Other |
|-------|------|----------|-----|-------|-------|
| _____ | _____ | | | | |
| _____ | _____ | | | | |

| LUNCH | Qty. | Calories | Fat | Carbs | Other |
|-------|------|----------|-----|-------|-------|
| _____ | _____ | | | | |
| _____ | _____ | | | | |
| _____ | _____ | | | | |
| _____ | _____ | | | | |
| _____ | _____ | | | | |

| SNACK | Qty. | Calories | Fat | Carbs | Other |
|-------|------|----------|-----|-------|-------|
| _____ | _____ | | | | |
| _____ | _____ | | | | |

| DINNER | Qty. | Calories | Fat | Carbs | Other |
|--------|------|----------|-----|-------|-------|
| _____ | _____ | | | | |
| _____ | _____ | | | | |
| _____ | _____ | | | | |
| _____ | _____ | | | | |
| _____ | _____ | | | | |

**DAILY INTAKE TOTALS:**

☑ **Water Intake**
# of 8 oz. glasses

☐ ☐ ☐
☐ ☐ ☐
☐ ☐ ☐

**Daily # of Servings**

fruits

veggies

grains

meats & beans

milk & dairy

oils & sweets

**Vitamins & Supplements:**

_____

_____

_____

_____

# FITNESS JOURNAL

DAILY GOAL: _____ GOAL MET: ☐

### CARDIOVASCULAR EXERCISE

| | Duration | Distance | Pace | Cal. Burned |
|---|---|---|---|---|
| | | | | |
| | | | | |
| | | | | |
| | | | | |

### STRENGTH TRAINING

| | Weight | Reps. | Sets | Cal. Burned |
|---|---|---|---|---|
| | | | | |
| | | | | |
| | | | | |
| | | | | |
| | | | | |
| | | | | |
| | | | | |
| | | | | |

### FLEXIBILITY, RELAXATION, MEDITATION

| | Duration | Cal. Burned |
|---|---|---|
| | | |
| | | |
| | | |

**DAILY CALORIES BURNED:**

---

### CALORIE CALCULATOR

| TOTAL CALORIE INTAKE | − | TOTAL CALORIES BURNED | = | NET CALORIES | − | BMR (Basal Metabolic Rate) | = | DAILY NET CALORIE GAIN OR LOSS |
|---|---|---|---|---|---|---|---|---|

**Energy Level:** 👎 1 2 3 4 5 6 👍

**Muscle Group Worked:** ☐ arms ☐ chest ☐ back ☐ core ☐ thighs ☐ calves

**Diet & Workout Notes:**

_____

_____

_____

_____

# Day 24

DATE: _____     WEIGHT: _____

| BREAKFAST | Qty. | Calories | Fat | Carbs | Other |
|-----------|------|----------|-----|-------|-------|
| _____ | _____ | | | | |
| _____ | _____ | | | | |
| _____ | _____ | | | | |
| _____ | _____ | | | | |
| _____ | _____ | | | | |

| SNACK | Qty. | Calories | Fat | Carbs | Other |
|-------|------|----------|-----|-------|-------|
| _____ | _____ | | | | |
| _____ | _____ | | | | |

| LUNCH | Qty. | Calories | Fat | Carbs | Other |
|-------|------|----------|-----|-------|-------|
| _____ | _____ | | | | |
| _____ | _____ | | | | |
| _____ | _____ | | | | |
| _____ | _____ | | | | |
| _____ | _____ | | | | |

| SNACK | Qty. | Calories | Fat | Carbs | Other |
|-------|------|----------|-----|-------|-------|
| _____ | _____ | | | | |
| _____ | _____ | | | | |

| DINNER | Qty. | Calories | Fat | Carbs | Other |
|--------|------|----------|-----|-------|-------|
| _____ | _____ | | | | |
| _____ | _____ | | | | |
| _____ | _____ | | | | |
| _____ | _____ | | | | |
| _____ | _____ | | | | |

**DAILY INTAKE TOTALS:**

☑ **Water Intake**
# of 8 oz. glasses

**Daily # of Servings**

| | fruits | | meats & beans |
| | veggies | | milk & dairy |
| | grains | | oils & sweets |

**Vitamins & Supplements:**
_____
_____
_____
_____

# FITNESS JOURNAL

**DAILY GOAL:** _____  **GOAL MET:** ☐

## CARDIOVASCULAR EXERCISE

| | Duration | Distance | Pace | Cal. Burned |
|---|---|---|---|---|
| _____ | | | | |
| _____ | | | | |
| _____ | | | | |
| _____ | | | | |

## STRENGTH TRAINING

| | Weight | Reps. | Sets | Cal. Burned |
|---|---|---|---|---|
| _____ | | | | |
| _____ | | | | |
| _____ | | | | |
| _____ | | | | |
| _____ | | | | |
| _____ | | | | |
| _____ | | | | |
| _____ | | | | |

## FLEXIBILITY, RELAXATION, MEDITATION

| | Duration | Cal. Burned |
|---|---|---|
| _____ | | |
| _____ | | |
| _____ | | |

**DAILY CALORIES BURNED:** _____

## CALORIE CALCULATOR

| | | | | |
|---|---|---|---|---|
| _____ − | _____ = | _____ − | _____ = | _____ |
| TOTAL CALORIE INTAKE | TOTAL CALORIES BURNED | NET CALORIES | BMR (Basal Metabolic Rate) | DAILY NET CALORIE GAIN OR LOSS |

**Energy Level:**  👎  1  2  3  4  5  6  👍

**Muscle Group Worked:**  ☐ arms  ☐ chest  ☐ back  ☐ core  ☐ thighs  ☐ calves

**Diet & Workout Notes:**

_____

_____

_____

_____

# Day 25

DATE:_____          WEIGHT:_____

**BREAKFAST** | Qty. | Calories | Fat | Carbs | Other
---|---|---|---|---|---

**SNACK** | Qty. | Calories | Fat | Carbs | Other
---|---|---|---|---|---

**LUNCH** | Qty. | Calories | Fat | Carbs | Other
---|---|---|---|---|---

**SNACK** | Qty. | Calories | Fat | Carbs | Other
---|---|---|---|---|---

**DINNER** | Qty. | Calories | Fat | Carbs | Other
---|---|---|---|---|---

**DAILY INTAKE TOTALS:**

☑ **Water Intake**
# of 8 oz. glasses

**Daily # of Servings**

fruits          meats & beans

veggies         milk & dairy

grains          oils & sweets

**Vitamins & Supplements:**

_____

_____

_____

_____

# FITNESS JOURNAL

DAILY GOAL: _____     GOAL MET: ☐

### 🏃 CARDIOVASCULAR EXERCISE

| | Duration | Distance | Pace | Cal. Burned |
|---|---|---|---|---|
| _____ | | | | |
| _____ | | | | |
| _____ | | | | |
| _____ | | | | |

### 🏋 STRENGTH TRAINING

| | Weight | Reps. | Sets | Cal. Burned |
|---|---|---|---|---|
| _____ | | | | |
| _____ | | | | |
| _____ | | | | |
| _____ | | | | |
| _____ | | | | |
| _____ | | | | |
| _____ | | | | |
| _____ | | | | |

### 方 FLEXIBILITY, RELAXATION, MEDITATION

| | Duration | Cal. Burned |
|---|---|---|
| _____ | | |
| _____ | | |
| _____ | | |

**DAILY CALORIES BURNED:** _____

---

### CALORIE CALCULATOR

| _____ | − | _____ | = | _____ | − | _____ | = | _____ |
|---|---|---|---|---|---|---|---|---|
| TOTAL CALORIE INTAKE | | TOTAL CALORIES BURNED | | NET CALORIES | | BMR (Basal Metabolic Rate) | | DAILY NET CALORIE GAIN OR LOSS |

---

**Energy Level:**
👎   1   2   3   4   5   6   👍

**Muscle Group Worked:**
☐ arms   ☐ chest   ☐ back   ☐ core   ☐ thighs   ☐ calves

**Diet & Workout Notes:**

_____

_____

_____

_____

# Day 26

DATE: _____          WEIGHT: _____

### 🍎 BREAKFAST

| | Qty. | Calories | Fat | Carbs | Other |
|---|---|---|---|---|---|
| _____ | _____ | | | | |
| _____ | _____ | | | | |
| _____ | _____ | | | | |
| _____ | _____ | | | | |
| _____ | _____ | | | | |

### 🍏 SNACK

| | Qty. | Calories | Fat | Carbs | Other |
|---|---|---|---|---|---|
| _____ | _____ | | | | |
| _____ | _____ | | | | |

### 🍔 LUNCH

| | Qty. | Calories | Fat | Carbs | Other |
|---|---|---|---|---|---|
| _____ | _____ | | | | |
| _____ | _____ | | | | |
| _____ | _____ | | | | |
| _____ | _____ | | | | |
| _____ | _____ | | | | |

### 🍇 SNACK

| | Qty. | Calories | Fat | Carbs | Other |
|---|---|---|---|---|---|
| _____ | _____ | | | | |
| _____ | _____ | | | | |

### 🥄 DINNER

| | Qty. | Calories | Fat | Carbs | Other |
|---|---|---|---|---|---|
| _____ | _____ | | | | |
| _____ | _____ | | | | |
| _____ | _____ | | | | |
| _____ | _____ | | | | |
| _____ | _____ | | | | |

**DAILY INTAKE TOTALS:**

☑ **Water Intake**
# of 8 oz. glasses

**Daily # of Servings**

| | fruits | | meats & beans |
| | veggies | | milk & dairy |
| | grains | | oils & sweets |

**Vitamins & Supplements:**

_____

_____

_____

# FITNESS JOURNAL

DAILY GOAL: _____     GOAL MET: ☐

## CARDIOVASCULAR EXERCISE

| | Duration | Distance | Pace | Cal. Burned |
|---|---|---|---|---|
| _____ | | | | |
| _____ | | | | |
| _____ | | | | |
| _____ | | | | |

## STRENGTH TRAINING

| | Weight | Reps. | Sets | Cal. Burned |
|---|---|---|---|---|
| _____ | | | | |
| _____ | | | | |
| _____ | | | | |
| _____ | | | | |
| _____ | | | | |
| _____ | | | | |
| _____ | | | | |
| _____ | | | | |

## FLEXIBILITY, RELAXATION, MEDITATION

| | Duration | Cal. Burned |
|---|---|---|
| _____ | | |
| _____ | | |
| _____ | | |

**DAILY CALORIES BURNED:** _____

### CALORIE CALCULATOR

| ____ | − | ____ | = | ____ | − | ____ | = | ____ |
|---|---|---|---|---|---|---|---|---|
| TOTAL CALORIE INTAKE | | TOTAL CALORIES BURNED | | NET CALORIES | | BMR (Basal Metabolic Rate) | | DAILY NET CALORIE GAIN OR LOSS |

**Energy Level:**  👎  1  2  3  4  5  6  👍

**Muscle Group Worked:** ☐ arms  ☐ chest  ☐ back  ☐ core  ☐ thighs  ☐ calves

**Diet & Workout Notes:**

_____

_____

_____

_____

# Day 27

DATE: _____          WEIGHT: _____

**BREAKFAST**      Qty.    Calories    Fat    Carbs    Other

**SNACK**      Qty.    Calories    Fat    Carbs    Other

**LUNCH**      Qty.    Calories    Fat    Carbs    Other

**SNACK**      Qty.    Calories    Fat    Carbs    Other

**DINNER**      Qty.    Calories    Fat    Carbs    Other

**DAILY INTAKE TOTALS:**

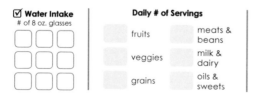

☑ **Water Intake**
# of 8 oz. glasses

**Daily # of Servings**

fruits

veggies

grains

meats & beans

milk & dairy

oils & sweets

**Vitamins & Supplements:**

# FITNESS JOURNAL

**DAILY GOAL:** _____  **GOAL MET:** ☐

### CARDIOVASCULAR EXERCISE

| | Duration | Distance | Pace | Cal. Burned |
|---|---|---|---|---|
| _____ | | | | |
| _____ | | | | |
| _____ | | | | |
| _____ | | | | |

### STRENGTH TRAINING

| | Weight | Reps. | Sets | Cal. Burned |
|---|---|---|---|---|
| _____ | | | | |
| _____ | | | | |
| _____ | | | | |
| _____ | | | | |
| _____ | | | | |
| _____ | | | | |
| _____ | | | | |
| _____ | | | | |

### FLEXIBILITY, RELAXATION, MEDITATION

| | Duration | Cal. Burned |
|---|---|---|
| _____ | | |
| _____ | | |
| _____ | | |

**DAILY CALORIES BURNED:** _____

## CALORIE CALCULATOR

| ____ − ____ = ____ − ____ = ____ |
|---|

| TOTAL CALORIE INTAKE | TOTAL CALORIES BURNED | NET CALORIES | BMR (Basal Metabolic Rate) | DAILY NET CALORIE GAIN OR LOSS |
|---|---|---|---|---|

**Energy Level:**   👎  1   2   3   4   5   6  👍

**Muscle Group Worked:**
☐ arms   ☐ chest   ☐ back   ☐ core   ☐ thighs   ☐ calves

**Diet & Workout Notes:**

_____

_____

_____

_____

# Day 28

DATE:_____    WEIGHT:_____

| BREAKFAST | Qty. | Calories | Fat | Carbs | Other |
|-----------|------|----------|-----|-------|-------|
| _____ | ____ | | | | |
| _____ | ____ | | | | |
| _____ | ____ | | | | |
| _____ | ____ | | | | |
| _____ | ____ | | | | |

| SNACK | Qty. | Calories | Fat | Carbs | Other |
|-------|------|----------|-----|-------|-------|
| _____ | ____ | | | | |
| _____ | ____ | | | | |

| LUNCH | Qty. | Calories | Fat | Carbs | Other |
|-------|------|----------|-----|-------|-------|
| _____ | ____ | | | | |
| _____ | ____ | | | | |
| _____ | ____ | | | | |
| _____ | ____ | | | | |
| _____ | ____ | | | | |

| SNACK | Qty. | Calories | Fat | Carbs | Other |
|-------|------|----------|-----|-------|-------|
| _____ | ____ | | | | |
| _____ | ____ | | | | |

| DINNER | Qty. | Calories | Fat | Carbs | Other |
|--------|------|----------|-----|-------|-------|
| _____ | ____ | | | | |
| _____ | ____ | | | | |
| _____ | ____ | | | | |
| _____ | ____ | | | | |
| _____ | ____ | | | | |

**DAILY INTAKE TOTALS:**

☑ **Water Intake**
# of 8 oz. glasses

**Daily # of Servings**

fruits          meats & beans

veggies        milk & dairy

grains          oils & sweets

**Vitamins & Supplements:**
_____
_____
_____
_____

# FITNESS JOURNAL

DAILY GOAL:_____    GOAL MET: ☐

### 🏃 CARDIOVASCULAR EXERCISE

| | Duration | Distance | Pace | Cal. Burned |
|---|---|---|---|---|
| | | | | |
| | | | | |
| | | | | |
| | | | | |

### 🏋 STRENGTH TRAINING

| | Weight | Reps. | Sets | Cal. Burned |
|---|---|---|---|---|
| | | | | |
| | | | | |
| | | | | |
| | | | | |
| | | | | |
| | | | | |
| | | | | |
| | | | | |

### 太 FLEXIBILITY, RELAXATION, MEDITATION

| | Duration | Cal. Burned |
|---|---|---|
| | | |
| | | |
| | | |

**DAILY CALORIES BURNED:** _____

---

## CALORIE CALCULATOR

| _____ | – | _____ | = | _____ | – | _____ | = | _____ |
|---|---|---|---|---|---|---|---|---|
| TOTAL CALORIE INTAKE | | TOTAL CALORIES BURNED | | NET CALORIES | | BMR (Basal Metabolic Rate) | | DAILY NET CALORIE GAIN OR LOSS |

**Energy Level:**
👎  1   2   3   4   5   6  👍

**Muscle Group Worked:**
☐ arms  ☐ chest  ☐ back  ☐ core  ☐ thighs  ☐ calves

**Diet & Workout Notes:**

_____
_____
_____
_____

# Day 29

DATE: _____     WEIGHT: _____

| BREAKFAST | Qty. | Calories | Fat | Carbs | Other |
|-----------|------|----------|-----|-------|-------|
| _____ | _____ | | | | |
| _____ | _____ | | | | |
| _____ | _____ | | | | |
| _____ | _____ | | | | |
| _____ | _____ | | | | |

| SNACK | Qty. | Calories | Fat | Carbs | Other |
|-------|------|----------|-----|-------|-------|
| _____ | _____ | | | | |
| _____ | _____ | | | | |

| LUNCH | Qty. | Calories | Fat | Carbs | Other |
|-------|------|----------|-----|-------|-------|
| _____ | _____ | | | | |
| _____ | _____ | | | | |
| _____ | _____ | | | | |
| _____ | _____ | | | | |
| _____ | _____ | | | | |

| SNACK | Qty. | Calories | Fat | Carbs | Other |
|-------|------|----------|-----|-------|-------|
| _____ | _____ | | | | |
| _____ | _____ | | | | |

| DINNER | Qty. | Calories | Fat | Carbs | Other |
|--------|------|----------|-----|-------|-------|
| _____ | _____ | | | | |
| _____ | _____ | | | | |
| _____ | _____ | | | | |
| _____ | _____ | | | | |
| _____ | _____ | | | | |

**DAILY INTAKE TOTALS:**

☑ **Water Intake**
# of 8 oz. glasses

**Daily # of Servings**

- fruits
- veggies
- grains
- meats & beans
- milk & dairy
- oils & sweets

**Vitamins & Supplements:**

_____
_____
_____

# FITNESS JOURNAL

DAILY GOAL: _____ GOAL MET: ☐

### CARDIOVASCULAR EXERCISE

| | Duration | Distance | Pace | Cal. Burned |
|---|---|---|---|---|
| | | | | |
| | | | | |
| | | | | |
| | | | | |

### STRENGTH TRAINING

| | Weight | Reps. | Sets | Cal. Burned |
|---|---|---|---|---|
| | | | | |
| | | | | |
| | | | | |
| | | | | |
| | | | | |
| | | | | |
| | | | | |
| | | | | |

### FLEXIBILITY, RELAXATION, MEDITATION

| | Duration | Cal. Burned |
|---|---|---|
| | | |
| | | |
| | | |

**DAILY CALORIES BURNED:**

## CALORIE CALCULATOR

|  | − |  | = |  | − |  | = |  |
|---|---|---|---|---|---|---|---|---|
| TOTAL CALORIE INTAKE | | TOTAL CALORIES BURNED | | NET CALORIES | | BMR (Basal Metabolic Rate) | | DAILY NET CALORIE GAIN OR LOSS |

**Energy Level:**  👎  1  2  3  4  5  6  👍

**Muscle Group Worked:** ☐ arms ☐ chest ☐ back ☐ core ☐ thighs ☐ calves

**Diet & Workout Notes:**

_____
_____
_____
_____

# Day 30

DATE: _____     WEIGHT: _____

| BREAKFAST | Qty. | Calories | Fat | Carbs | Other |
|-----------|------|----------|-----|-------|-------|
| | | | | | |
| | | | | | |
| | | | | | |
| | | | | | |
| | | | | | |

| SNACK | Qty. | Calories | Fat | Carbs | Other |
|-------|------|----------|-----|-------|-------|
| | | | | | |
| | | | | | |

| LUNCH | Qty. | Calories | Fat | Carbs | Other |
|-------|------|----------|-----|-------|-------|
| | | | | | |
| | | | | | |
| | | | | | |
| | | | | | |
| | | | | | |

| SNACK | Qty. | Calories | Fat | Carbs | Other |
|-------|------|----------|-----|-------|-------|
| | | | | | |
| | | | | | |

| DINNER | Qty. | Calories | Fat | Carbs | Other |
|--------|------|----------|-----|-------|-------|
| | | | | | |
| | | | | | |
| | | | | | |
| | | | | | |
| | | | | | |

**DAILY INTAKE TOTALS:**

☑ **Water Intake**
# of 8 oz. glasses

**Daily # of Servings**

fruits      meats & beans
veggies     milk & dairy
grains      oils & sweets

**Vitamins & Supplements:**
_____
_____
_____
_____

# FITNESS JOURNAL

DAILY GOAL: _____     GOAL MET: ☐

### 🏃 CARDIOVASCULAR EXERCISE

| | Duration | Distance | Pace | Cal. Burned |
|---|---|---|---|---|
| _____ | | | | |
| _____ | | | | |
| _____ | | | | |
| _____ | | | | |

### 🏋 STRENGTH TRAINING

| | Weight | Reps. | Sets | Cal. Burned |
|---|---|---|---|---|
| _____ | | | | |
| _____ | | | | |
| _____ | | | | |
| _____ | | | | |
| _____ | | | | |
| _____ | | | | |
| _____ | | | | |
| _____ | | | | |

### 🧘 FLEXIBILITY, RELAXATION, MEDITATION

| | Duration | Cal. Burned |
|---|---|---|
| _____ | | |
| _____ | | |
| _____ | | |

**DAILY CALORIES BURNED:** _____

---

## CALORIE CALCULATOR

| [____] | − | [____] | = | [____] | − | [____] | = | [____] |
|---|---|---|---|---|---|---|---|---|
| TOTAL CALORIE INTAKE | | TOTAL CALORIES BURNED | | NET CALORIES | | BMR (Basal Metabolic Rate) | | DAILY NET CALORIE GAIN OR LOSS |

**Energy Level:** 👎 **1  2  3  4  5  6** 👍

**Muscle Group Worked:** ☐ arms  ☐ chest  ☐ back  ☐ core  ☐ thighs  ☐ calves

**Diet & Workout Notes:**

_____
_____
_____
_____

# 18

"Whether you think you can or think you can't
— you are right."
~ Henry Ford

# Maintaining Your Weight Loss

**Congratulations, you made it through the program!** But what happens now? This chapter is going to cover the ways to maintain your weight loss and continue to lose even more weight — but first, you should celebrate your weight-loss accomplishments! Remember, use what you've learned in this book and celebrate without bingeing or indulging in a high-calorie meal. Healthy celebrations include going to a concert or sporting event, seeing a movie with a loved one, shopping for a new item of clothing to fit your slimmed-down shape, or treating yourself to a kitchen appliance you've had your eye on. If the reward helps you continue to lose weight, even better!

After you've sufficiently rewarded yourself for a job well done, it's time to think long-term. Do you want to continue losing weight with this diet and fitness program? Well, why not? If you followed the food and exercise tips, tricks, and secrets here you lost weight and inches in a short amount of time without feeling stressed, starved, or deprived. And after a few weeks, these behaviors have had enough time to become real habits and lifestyle changes. So why stop now?

There are a few things to be aware of, however. For one, you may hit a point where your weight loss slows down from 1 or 2 pounds per week to less than 1 pound. You may even hit a plateau and stop losing weight all together. This is perfectly normal. Your body is slimming down, you have less weight and body fat to lose, and you are growing accustomed to eating less and exercising more. Consider getting a trainer who can help you mix up your routine, use new machines, and try new techniques you may never have considered. When you do the same exercises or strength training workout, you're firing the same muscle fibers again and again — and they begin to adapt. You may also need to work out longer to keep losing weight. But don't worry — as you build muscle and lose fat, your body will automatically burn more calories when it's at rest.

But truly, the greatest thing you'll find about the *Lose Weight Fast Diet* program is that exercising and eating right become a way of life! Plopping down on the couch with a bag of chips won't seem appealing to you anymore. And your body will have become used to eating smaller meals, so pigging out on half a pizza won't be on your mind.

Just don't lose your focus, stop watching your portion sizes, or get lazy with exercise. Read on for some great ways to enjoy your success but keep losing weight while sticking to your new, healthy, happy lifestyle.

## Start thinking of yourself as thin

Sadly, many people who slim down still view themselves as their former, larger selves. They wear the same clothes they wore when they were heavier or save a place in their closets for their "fat" clothes. Many overweight people shy away from wearing bright colors that draw attention to problem areas and still end up dressing in all black after they lose weight. But now is the time to embrace change and show off your hard work! Invest in a few new pieces and feel proud wearing them. Not only are you rewarding yourself, you'll look better too. Wearing clothing that is too big for you isn't flattering and will only hide your flatter stomach and more defined arms and legs. And do some closet spring cleaning too. Anything dowdy, oversized, or out of shape can be donated to charity. Some people hold on to all their old clothes because they're afraid they'll gain the weight back, but getting rid of them means you're saying goodbye to the old you who sat on the couch with a bowl of ice cream every night. This new you exercises, eats right throughout the week, and celebrates a healthy, thinner figure. Just don't go on a shopping spree if you're planning to lose more weight (and you should be!). Wait until you're down 2 full sizes to splurge on a new wardrobe.

## Revamp your daily routine to include fitness

So how many days a week are you going to need to exercise to maintain or increase your weight loss after you've completed this program? Consider that the men and women of the National Weight Control Registry (a roster of more than 6,000 participants who, on average, have lost 66 pounds and kept them off for 5 ½ years), report exercising for an average of 60 to 75 minutes daily. If you are not the type of person who enjoys going to a gym you'll need to integrate other forms of calorie-burning activities into your life. For instance, vacuuming for one hour burns 220 calories, grocery shopping requires 180 calories, and an afternoon of gardening, sweeping and raking leaves expends 270 calories. If your home or office has stairs, walking up them in a moderate manner for 15 minutes burns 120 calories. Need a room in your house painted? Do it yourself and burn 340 calories an hour. Live in an area with snow? You've hit the jackpot — shoveling snow for an hour burns 600 calories. Combining a few of these forms of aerobic activity is the equivalent of spending a couple of hours at the gym.

## Make new friends who also care about healthy living

If you've joined a gym or fitness class or group, you have ample opportunities to make new friends, and the best part is, these are people who care about being healthy and staying slim too. Losing weight often opens doors to more confidence and many times, a new social life. Accept more invitations to parties and get-togethers; wear something that makes you feel amazing and that shows off your hard work. Being around people who share your interest in eating well and being healthy, as well as people who praise your weight loss, will keep you motivated to keep working hard.

## Must have a treat? Keep it reasonable

If you really want to enjoy a treat in the form of food, keep it under 250 calories. A small sundae or miniature cupcake will do the trick. Just consciously remind yourself that this is a treat at the end of your hard work and not an invitation to go back to your old bad habits. This is a one-time celebration and not a weekly event.

## Beat the weight-loss plateau

Naturally, the same diet and workout aren't going to produce the same results week after week. There are many ways to break through the plateaus you'll inevitably encounter. Let's say you have been doing cardio 5 days a week for 45 minutes; either add an extra 15 minutes to a few workouts, or else turn a normal session into an interval session just by interspersing 30- to 60-second bursts of speed and intensity every few minutes. Or break through a plateau by changing up your meal routine. For instance, try eating a bigger lunch with more fiber and a smaller dinner. This can help take advantage of when your metabolism is faster during the day.

## Document your progress with photos and measurements

The scale may not always accurately reflect your weight loss, considering that muscle greatly outweighs fat, and that water weight can be a factor as well. The best way to document your progress is with photos (take them in a similar swimsuit each time) and by measuring yourself around the hips, thighs, stomach, chest, and arms. Losing inches (as well as pants and dress sizes) are the true test of your weight-loss success. And seeing your new, slimmer self reflected in photos is one of the best testaments to how well this program has worked for you. When you feel like giving up or going back to your old ways, you can look at your "Before" and "After" photos and feel fantastic about how far you've come, and how much weight you've lost all over. This confidence and pride are what keeps you going.

## Stave off boredom

One common excuse for abandoning a workout or weight-loss program is boredom. Naturally, people get sick of the same gym grind or meal plan. When boredom starts to threaten your weight loss, it's time to introduce a new form of exercise or try one that never gets dull. Yoga, for instance, is a fantastic full-body workout and is a practice that is ever-evolving. Because there's always a new level of intensity or difficulty to reach, your body will never get complacent and you won't get bored. Or try taking up something that takes a long time to master, such as surfing, which is another great full-body workout — and fun, too!

The same concept goes for the foods you eat as well. Although a minority of people say they like the routine of eating the same thing at every meal, most people get bored and eventually succumb to cravings. Change up your go-to low-calorie meals in easy ways. Swap grilled salmon for chicken in a salad; add shredded chicken and avocado to a bowl of soup; experiment with a new vegetable on the side of your dinner.

## Update your music playlist every month

Music inspires you to get moving and keep moving. A great playlist keeps your energy up, but, just like anything, you will get bored if you're listening to the same songs day in and day out. It's a great idea to make separate playlists for different workouts of varying intensities; for example, a super-fast set of songs for running, interval training and weight lifting, a slower set for jogging, and a relaxing, calming set for stretching and cooling down. Try varying the songs on each playlist every month. Check on your local radio stations' websites for what's new, or visit ShapeMagazine.com — they offer great monthly playlists for up-tempo workouts, and you can click right through to purchase the songs on iTunes.

## Calculate your new daily calorie allowance

Now that you've lost weight, you may be ready to simply maintain your weight, or you may be interested in losing even more. To do that, you need to calculate your new BMR (it changes as you lose weight) and new daily calorie allowance. That is the number of calories you'd need to eat each day to maintain your current weight. If you want to lose more weight, you should create another calorie deficit, in the same way you did throughout this program.

The following equation uses your new BMR and factors in activity level:

To calculate your new BMR:

Women BMR = 655 + (4.3 x weight in pounds) + (4.7 x height in inches) - (4.7 x age in years)

Men BMR = 66 + (6.3 x weight in pounds) + (12.9 x height in inches) - (6.8 x age in years)

To find daily calorie allowance, choose the appropriate activity level and ·
multiply your BMR accordingly.

Sedentary (little or no exercise):

**Calorie-Calculation = BMR x 1.2**

Lightly active (light exercise/activity 1-3 days/week):

**Calorie-Calculation = BMR x 1.375**

Moderately active (moderate exercise/activity 3-5 days/week):

**Calorie-Calculation = BMR x 1.55**

Very active (hard exercise/activity 6-7 days a week):

**Calorie-Calculation = BMR x 1.725**

Extra active (very hard exercise/activity, physical job or sports
conditioning):

**Calorie-Calculation = BMR x 1.9**

The result of this calculation is the number of calories you can eat every
day and maintain your current weight. If you want to lose more weight,
reduce your calories to a number below your maintenance level. Just keep
in mind, according to the American College of Sports Medicine, calorie
intake should never drop below 1,200 calories per day for women or 1,800
calories per day for men. Even those amounts are incredibly low. Keep
your calories at a level that allows you to feel full and gives you enough
energy for exercise.

## Do what works for others

In observing National Weight Control Registry members, it is important to determine how they manage to keep the weight off when such a huge majority of dieters fail to do so. In the end, there are 3 main factors that members continue to report again and again, which this book has already highlighted. Stick with these moving forward, and you're sure to keep the weight off and lose even more. In order to maintain their weight loss, NWCR members:

- 78% eat breakfast every day
- 62% watch less than 10 hours of TV per week
- 90% exercise, on average, about 1 hour per day

## Get your family and friends involved in your new lifestyle

The only way to maintain this new, healthier way of life is to get the people closest to you onboard as well. That means being active with your family and friends. If you have kids, take up an activity that you can all do together, such as horseback riding, skiing, cycling, surfing, or even yoga. If you have very young children, a game of tag is enough to get you all active and moving together.

Invite your friends to be active with you as well. Most people will be excited and willing to try a new activity with you, especially if they have witnessed your weight-loss success firsthand.

Your family and friends should also join you in your efforts to eat low-calorie, low-fat meals as often as possible. Try adding shredded vegetables, such as carrots, squash, or zucchini into pasta sauces, or substituting meatless products into entrées like burritos and omelets — your fellow diners will never know the difference! Serve healthy desserts, such as fresh fruit with low-fat whipped topping, and your family will start to crave the same healthy foods that are helping you lose weight.

## Don't stop using a diet and fitness journal!

Losing weight is one thing, but keeping it off is another. Unfortunately, most people who successfully lose weight end up putting it (plus more) back on. A government review of numerous weight-loss studies found that two-thirds of dieters gain all the weight back within a year. But why does it happen and how can you avoid being part of that statistic?

For one, people get lazy once they've lost weight. They stop doing what worked for them. They stop monitoring their portion sizes and stop updating a food and fitness journal. Don't forget how easy it is for the calories from a handful of M&M's at work or finishing your child's hotdog at a baseball game to creep in.

Don't stop writing in your diet and fitness journal just because this program is over. You can easily continue using the same secrets and methods for losing even more weight. Be sure to get a new journal before you've completely filled out the 4 weeks of journal pages in this book — that way you won't miss a day! Try the *Lose Weight Fast Diet Journal*, the companion journal to this book, and one of the best-selling titles on the market. Also, you should keep a calorie-counting tool handy for when you dine out and eateries don't offer nutritional information. A great book is the portable, pocket-size *Complete Calorie, Fat & Carb Counter*, which provides calories, fat, carbs, fiber, and protein for menu items from more than 500 fast food chains, restaurants, and popular food brands.

Studies have shown again and again that keeping a diet and workout journal is one of the most effective tools for weight loss there is. Your success with this program should have confirmed that fact for you with your new and improved body. So don't stop making great choices and writing them down!

# Chapter 19

"Knowledge comes by eyes always open and working hands; and there is no knowledge that is not power."

~ Ralph Waldo Emerson

# Nutrition Facts

This section is a great resource for nutritional information on foods you may want to select for your fitness and weight-loss program. It provides calories per serving, as well as the content in grams for fat, protein, carbohydrates, and fiber.

To use this section, look up a food item and its corresponding information. Then log this data in your journal so that you can track your daily totals.

# NUTRITION FACTS

| FOOD ITEM | Serving Size | Cal | Fat | Cbs | Prtn | Fbr |
|---|---|---|---|---|---|---|
| **A** | | | | | | |
| Alcohol, 100 proof | 1 fl.oz. | 82 | 0 | 0 | 0 | 0 |
| Alcohol, 86 proof | 1 fl.oz. | 70 | 0 | 0 | 0 | 0 |
| Alcohol, 90 proof | 1 fl.oz. | 73 | 0 | 0 | 0 | 0 |
| Alcohol, 94 proof | 1 fl.oz. | 76 | 0 | 0 | 0 | 0 |
| Alcohol, dessert wine, dry | 1 glass | 157 | 0 | 12 | 0 | 0 |
| Alcohol, dessert wine, sweet | 1 glass | 165 | 0 | 14 | 0 | 0 |
| Alcohol, liquors | 1 fl.oz. | 107 | 0 | 11 | 0 | 0 |
| Alcohol, pina colada | 8 fl.oz. | 440 | 5 | 57 | 1 | 0 |
| Alfalfa seeds | 1 tbsp | 1 | 0 | 0 | 0 | 0 |
| Allspice, ground | 1 tsp | 5 | 0 | 1 | 0 | 0 |
| Almond butter, w/ salt | 1 tbsp | 101 | 10 | 3 | 2 | 1 |
| Almond butter, w/o salt | 1 tbsp | 101 | 10 | 3 | 2 | 1 |
| Almonds, roasted | 1 oz. (12 nuts) | 169 | 15 | 6 | 6 | 3 |
| Anchovies | 3 oz. | 111 | 4 | 0 | 17 | 0 |
| Apple cider, powdered | 1 packet | 83 | 0 | 21 | 0 | 0 |
| Apple juice | 8 fl.oz. | 120 | 0 | 29 | 0 | 0 |
| Apples, w/o skin | 1 medium | 61 | 0 | 16 | 0 | 2 |
| Apples, w/ skin | 1 medium | 72 | 0 | 19 | 0 | 3 |
| Applesauce | 1 cup | 194 | 1 | 51 | 1 | 3 |
| Apricots | 1 apricot | 17 | 0 | 4 | 1 | 1 |
| Arrowroot | 1 cup, sliced | 78 | 0 | 16 | 5 | 2 |
| Arrowroot flour | 1 cup | 457 | 0 | 113 | 0 | 4 |
| Artichokes | 1 artichoke | 76 | 0 | 17 | 5 | 9 |
| Arugula | 1 cup | 4 | 0 | 1 | 1 | 0 |
| Asparagus | 1 spear | 2 | 0 | 1 | 0 | 0 |
| Avocados | 1 cup, cubes | 240 | 22 | 13 | 3 | 10 |
| **B** | | | | | | |
| Bacon bits, meatless | 1 tbsp | 33 | 2 | 2 | 2 | 1 |
| Bacon, canadian, cooked | 1 slice | 43 | 2 | 0 | 6 | 0 |
| Bacon, meatless | 1 slice | 16 | 2 | 0 | 1 | 0 |
| Bacon, pork, cooked | 1 slice | 42 | 3 | 0 | 3 | 0 |
| Bagels, cinnamon-raisin | 1 bagel, 4" dia | 244 | 2 | 49 | 9 | 2 |
| Bagels, egg | 1 bagel, 4" dia | 292 | 2 | 56 | 11 | 2 |
| Bagels, oat-bran | 1 bagel, 4" dia | 227 | 1 | 47 | 10 | 3 |
| Bagels, plain | 1 bagel, 4" dia | 245 | 1 | 47 | 9 | 2 |
| Bagels, deli gourmet style | 1 bagel | 370 | 3 | 71 | 13 | 2 |
| Balsam pear | 1 balsam pear | 21 | 0 | 5 | 1 | 4 |
| Bamboo shoots | 1 cup | 41 | 1 | 8 | 4 | 3 |
| Banana chips | 1 oz. | 147 | 10 | 17 | 1 | 2 |

Nutrition values for fat, carbohydrates (Cbs), protein (Prtn), and fiber (Fbr)
are listed in grams per serving. Serving sizes and values are approximate.

| FOOD ITEM | Serving Size | Cal | Fat | Cbs | Prtn | Fbr |
|---|---|---|---|---|---|---|
| **B (cont.)** | | | | | | |
| Bananas | 1 medium, 7"-8" | 105 | 0 | 27 | 1 | 3 |
| Barley | 1 cup | 651 | 4 | 135 | 23 | 32 |
| Barley flour | 1 cup | 511 | 2 | 110 | 16 | 15 |
| Barley, pearled, cooked | 1 cup | 193 | 1 | 44 | 4 | 6 |
| Basil | 5 leaves | 1 | 0 | 0 | 0 | 0 |
| Basil, dried | 1 tsp | 2 | 0 | 0 | 0 | 0 |
| Bay leaf | 1 tsp, crumbled | 2 | 0 | 0 | 0 | 0 |
| Beans, adzuki, cooked | 1 cup | 294 | 0 | 57 | 17 | 17 |
| Beans, baked, canned, plain | 1 cup | 239 | 1 | 54 | 12 | 10 |
| Beans, baked, canned, w/o salt | 1 cup | 266 | 1 | 52 | 12 | 13 |
| Beans, baked, canned, w/ beef | 1 cup | 322 | 9 | 54 | 17 | 10 |
| Beans, black, cooked | 1 cup | 227 | 1 | 40 | 15 | 15 |
| Beans, cranberry, cooked | 1 cup | 241 | 1 | 43 | 16 | 18 |
| Beans, fava, canned | 1 cup | 182 | 1 | 31 | 14 | 10 |
| Beans, french, cooked | 1 cup | 228 | 1 | 43 | 12 | 17 |
| Beans, great northern, cooked | 1 cup | 209 | 1 | 37 | 15 | 12 |
| Beans, kidney, cooked | 1 cup | 225 | 1 | 40 | 15 | 11 |
| Beans, lima, cooked | 1 cup | 216 | 1 | 39 | 15 | 13 |
| Beans, lima, canned | 1 can | 190 | 0 | 36 | 12 | 11 |
| Beans, mung, cooked | 1 cup | 212 | 1 | 39 | 14 | 15 |
| Beans, mungo, cooked | 1 cup | 189 | 1 | 33 | 14 | 12 |
| Beans, navy, cooked | 1 cup | 255 | 1 | 47 | 15 | 19 |
| Beans, pink, cooked | 1 cup | 252 | 1 | 47 | 15 | 9 |
| Beans, pinto, cooked | 1 cup | 245 | 1 | 44 | 15 | 15 |
| Beans, small white, cooked | 1 cup | 254 | 1 | 46 | 16 | 18 |
| Beans, snap, green, cooked | 1 cup | 44 | 0 | 10 | 2 | 4 |
| Beans, snap, yellow, cooked | 1 cup | 44 | 0 | 10 | 2 | 4 |
| Beans, white, cooked | 1 cup | 249 | 1 | 45 | 17 | 11 |
| Beans, yellow | 1 cup | 255 | 2 | 48 | 16 | 18 |
| Beechnuts, dried | 1 oz. | 163 | 14 | 10 | 2 | 0 |
| Beef, choice short rib, cooked | 3 oz. | 400 | 36 | 0 | 18 | 0 |
| Beef bologna | 1 slice | 88 | 8 | 1 | 3 | 0 |
| Beef jerky, chopped | 1 piece | 81 | 5 | 2 | 7 | 0 |
| Beef sausage, precooked | 1 link | 134 | 12 | 1 | 6 | 0 |
| Beef stew, canned | 1 serving | 218 | 13 | 16 | 12 | 4 |
| Beef, tri-tip roast, roasted | 3 oz. | 174 | 9 | 0 | 22 | 0 |
| Beef, brisket, lean and fat, roasted | 3 oz. | 328 | 27 | 0 | 20 | 0 |
| Beef, brisket, lean, roasted | 3 oz. | 206 | 11 | 0 | 25 | 0 |
| Beef, chuck, arm roast, lean & fat, braised | 3 oz. | 283 | 20 | 0 | 23 | 0 |
| Beef, chuck, arm roast, lean, braised | 3 oz. | 179 | 7 | 0 | 28 | 0 |

Nutrition values for fat, carbohydrates (Cbs), protein (Prtn), and fiber (Fbr)
are listed in grams per serving. Serving sizes and values are approximate.

| FOOD ITEM | Serving Size | Cal | Fat | Cbs | Prtn | Fbr |
|---|---|---|---|---|---|---|
| **B (cont.)** | | | | | | |
| Beef, chuck, top blade, raw | 3 oz. | 138 | 8 | 0 | 17 | 0 |
| Beef, cured breakfast strips | 3 slices | 276 | 26 | 1 | 9 | 0 |
| Beef, cured, corned, canned | 3 oz. | 213 | 13 | 0 | 23 | 0 |
| Beef, cured, dried | 1 serving | 43 | 1 | 1 | 9 | 0 |
| Beef, cured, luncheon meat | 1 slice | 31 | 1 | 0 | 5 | 0 |
| Beef, flank, raw | 1 oz. | 47 | 2 | 0 | 6 | 0 |
| Beef, ground patties, frozen | 3 oz. | 240 | 20 | 0 | 15 | 0 |
| Beef, ground, 70% lean, raw | 1 oz. | 94 | 9 | 0 | 4 | 0 |
| Beef, ground, 80% lean, raw | 1 oz. | 72 | 6 | 0 | 5 | 0 |
| Beef, ground, 95% lean, raw | 1 oz. | 39 | 1 | 0 | 6 | 0 |
| Beef, rib, large end, boneless, raw | 1 oz. | 94 | 8 | 0 | 5 | 0 |
| Beef, rib, shortribs, boneless, raw | 1 oz. | 110 | 10 | 0 | 4 | 0 |
| Beef, rib, whole, boneless, raw | 1 oz. | 91 | 8 | 0 | 5 | 0 |
| Beef, rib-eye, small end, raw | 1 oz. | 78 | 6 | 0 | 5 | 0 |
| Beef, round, bottom, raw | 1 oz. | 56 | 3 | 0 | 6 | 0 |
| Beef, round, eye, raw | 1 oz. | 49 | 3 | 0 | 6 | 0 |
| Beef, round, full cut, raw | 1 oz. | 55 | 3 | 0 | 6 | 0 |
| Beef, round, tip, raw | 1 oz. | 56 | 4 | 0 | 6 | 0 |
| Beef, round, top, raw | 1 oz. | 48 | 2 | 0 | 6 | 0 |
| Beef, shank crosscuts, raw | 1 oz. | 50 | 3 | 0 | 6 | 0 |
| Beef, short loin, porterhouse, raw | 1 oz. | 73 | 6 | 0 | 5 | 0 |
| Beef, short loin, t-bone, raw | 1 oz. | 66 | 5 | 0 | 5 | 0 |
| Beef, short loin, top, raw | 1 oz. | 66 | 5 | 0 | 6 | 0 |
| Beef, sirloin, tri-tip, raw | 1 oz. | 50 | 3 | 0 | 6 | 0 |
| Beef, tenderloin, raw | 1 oz. | 70 | 5 | 0 | 6 | 0 |
| Beef, top sirloin, raw | 1 oz. | 61 | 4 | 0 | 6 | 0 |
| Beer, light | 12 fl.oz. | 110 | 0 | 6 | 0 | 0 |
| Beer, nonalcoholic | 12 fl.oz. | 80 | 0 | 15 | 0 | 0 |
| Beer, regular | 12 fl.oz. | 140 | 0 | 12 | 0 | 0 |
| Beets | 1 beet | 35 | 0 | 8 | 2 | 4 |
| Bratwurst, chicken | 1 serving | 148 | 9 | 0 | 16 | 0 |
| Bratwurst, pork | 1 serving | 281 | 25 | 2 | 12 | 0 |
| Bratwurst, veal | 1 serving | 286 | 27 | 0 | 12 | 0 |
| Bread stuffing, dry mix, prepared | 1/2 cup | 178 | 9 | 22 | 3 | 3 |
| Bread, banana | 1 slice | 196 | 6 | 33 | 3 | 1 |
| Bread, corn | 1 piece | 188 | 6 | 29 | 4 | 1 |
| Bread, cracked-wheat | 1 slice | 65 | 1 | 12 | 2 | 1 |
| Bread, french | 1 slice | 70 | 1 | 15 | 3 | 1 |
| Bread, garlic | 1 slice | 160 | 10 | 14 | 3 | 1 |
| Bread, Irish soda | 1 oz. | 82 | 1 | 16 | 2 | 1 |

Nutrition values for fat, carbohydrates (Cbs), protein (Prtn), and fiber (Fbr) are listed in grams per serving. Serving sizes and values are approximate.

| FOOD ITEM | Serving Size | Cal | Fat | Cbs | Prtn | Fbr |
|---|---|---|---|---|---|---|
| **B (cont.)** | | | | | | |
| Bread, pita | 2 oz. | 150 | 1 | 30 | 3 | 0 |
| Bread, pumpernickel | 1 slice | 75 | 1 | 15 | 3 | 2 |
| Bread, raisin | 1 slice | 80 | 2 | 15 | 2 | 1 |
| Bread, rice bran | 1 oz. | 69 | 1 | 12 | 3 | 1 |
| Bread, sandwich slice | 1 slice | 70 | 1 | 13 | 2 | 1 |
| Bread, sourdough | 1 slice | 100 | 1 | 20 | 2 | 1 |
| Broad beans, cooked | 1 cup | 187 | 1 | 33 | 13 | 9 |
| Brownies | 1 brownie | 220 | 13 | 27 | 1 | 1 |
| Buckwheat | 1 cup | 583 | 6 | 122 | 23 | 17 |
| Buckwheat flour | 1 cup | 402 | 4 | 85 | 15 | 12 |
| Buckwheat groats, roasted, cooked | 1 cup | 155 | 1 | 34 | 6 | 5 |
| Buffalo, raw | 1 oz. | 28 | 0 | 0 | 6 | 0 |
| Burbot, raw | 3 oz. | 77 | 1 | 0 | 16 | 0 |
| Burdock root | 1 cup | 85 | 0 | 21 | 2 | 4 |
| Butter, whipped, w/ salt | 1 tbsp | 67 | 8 | 0 | 0 | 0 |
| Butternuts, dried | 1 oz. | 174 | 16 | 3 | 7 | 1 |
| | | | | | | |
| **C** | | | | | | |
| Cabbage, common | 1 cup, shredded | 17 | 1 | 4 | 1 | 2 |
| Cabbage, pak choi | 1 cup, shredded | 9 | 0 | 2 | 1 | 1 |
| Cabbage, pe-tsai | 1 cup, shredded | 12 | 0 | 3 | 1 | 1 |
| Cake, angel food | 1 slice | 180 | 4 | 36 | 2 | 2 |
| Cake, boston cream pie | 1 slice | 260 | 9 | 32 | 1 | 0 |
| Cake, carrot | 1 slice | 310 | 16 | 39 | 1 | 0 |
| Cake, cheesecake | 1 slice | 500 | 30 | 50 | 4 | 0 |
| Cake, chocolate | 1 slice | 270 | 13 | 36 | 1 | 1 |
| Cake, chocolate mousse | 1 slice | 250 | 10 | 35 | 1 | 1 |
| Cake, devil's food | 1 slice | 270 | 13 | 35 | 2 | 0 |
| Cake, pineapple upside-down | 1 piece | 367 | 14 | 58 | 4 | 1 |
| Cake, pound | 1 slice | 320 | 16 | 38 | 2 | 0 |
| Cake, sponge cake w/ cream, berries | 1 slice | 325 | 8 | 38 | 25 | 1 |
| Cake, yellow | 1 slice | 260 | 11 | 36 | 2 | 1 |
| Candy, butterscotch | 5 pieces | 120 | 3 | 20 | 0 | 0 |
| Candy, caramels | 1 piece | 30 | 1 | 6 | 3 | 1 |
| Candy, carob | 1 bar | 470 | 27 | 49 | 7 | 3 |
| Candy, chocolate fudge | 1 oz. | 125 | 5 | 18 | 0 | 0 |
| Candy, chocolate mints | 1 mint | 45 | 1 | 9 | 0 | 0 |
| Candy, milk chocolate w/ almonds | 2 oz. | 216 | 14 | 21 | 4 | 3 |
| Candy, chocolate-coated peanut butter bites | 1 piece | 45 | 3 | 4 | 1 | 0 |
| Candy, chocolate-coated peanuts | 12 peanuts | 160 | 11 | 15 | 20 | 7 |

Nutrition values for fat, carbohydrates (Cbs), protein (Prtn), and fiber (Fbr) are listed in grams per serving. Serving sizes and values are approximate.

# NUTRITION FACTS

| FOOD ITEM | Serving Size | Cal | Fat | Cbs | Prtn | Fbr |
|---|---|---|---|---|---|---|
| **C (cont.)** | | | | | | |
| Candy, gumdrops | 4 pieces | 130 | 0 | 31 | 0 | 0 |
| Candy, hard candy | 1 piece | 18 | 0 | 5 | 0 | 0 |
| Candy, jelly beans | 12 beans | 100 | 0 | 24 | 0 | 0 |
| Candy, licorice | 1 piece | 30 | 0 | 7 | 0 | 0 |
| Candy, lollipop | 1 lollipop | 20 | 0 | 5 | 0 | 0 |
| Candy, milk chocolate bar | 2 oz. | 235 | 13 | 26 | 3 | 2 |
| Candy, mints | 1 mint | 30 | 0 | 7 | 0 | 0 |
| Cantaloupe | 1 cup, cubed | 54 | 0 | 13 | 1 | 1 |
| Cardoon | 1 cup, shredded | 36 | 0 | 9 | 1 | 3 |
| Carrots | 1 medium | 65 | 0 | 15 | 1 | 4 |
| Cashew butter, w/ salt | 1 tbsp | 94 | 8 | 4 | 3 | 0 |
| Cashew nuts | 1 oz. | 157 | 12 | 9 | 5 | 1 |
| Cassava | 1 cup | 330 | 1 | 78 | 3 | 4 |
| Celeriac | 1 cup | 66 | 1 | 14 | 2 | 3 |
| Chard, swiss | 1 cup | 7 | 0 | 1 | 1 | 1 |
| Cheese, american | 1 slice | 50 | 3 | 2 | 4 | 0 |
| Cheese, brick | 1 oz. | 100 | 8 | 0 | 7 | 0 |
| Cheese, brie | 1 oz. | 95 | 8 | 1 | 5 | 0 |
| Cheese, camembert | 1 oz. | 90 | 7 | 1 | 5 | 0 |
| Cheese, cheddar | 1 oz. | 110 | 9 | 1 | 7 | 0 |
| Cheese, colby jack | 1 oz. | 110 | 9 | 1 | 7 | 0 |
| Cheese, cottage, 2% | 1 cup | 203 | 4 | 8 | 31 | 0 |
| Cheese, edam | 1 oz. | 100 | 8 | 0 | 7 | 0 |
| Cheese, feta | 1 oz. | 75 | 6 | 1 | 4 | 0 |
| Cheese, goat | 1 oz. | 128 | 10 | 1 | 9 | 0 |
| Cheese, goat, semisoft | 1 oz. | 103 | 9 | 1 | 6 | 0 |
| Cheese, goat, soft | 1 oz. | 76 | 6 | 0 | 5 | 0 |
| Cheese, gouda | 1 oz. | 100 | 8 | 1 | 7 | 0 |
| Cheese, monterey jack | 1 oz. | 110 | 9 | 0 | 7 | 0 |
| Cheese, mozzarella | 1 oz. | 90 | 7 | 1 | 6 | 0 |
| Cheese, parmesan, hard | 1 oz. | 110 | 7 | 1 | 10 | 0 |
| Cheese, parmesan, shredded | 1 tbsp | 22 | 2 | 0 | 2 | 0 |
| Cheese, provolone | 1 oz. | 100 | 8 | 1 | 7 | 0 |
| Cheese, queso | 2 tbsp | 110 | 9 | 2 | 6 | 0 |
| Cheese, ricotta | 2 tbsp | 50 | 4 | 1 | 4 | 0 |
| Cheese, roquefort | 1 oz. | 105 | 9 | 1 | 6 | 0 |
| Cheese, swiss | 1 oz. | 110 | 9 | 1 | 8 | 0 |
| Cherries, sour | 8 pieces | 30 | 0 | 7 | 1 | 2 |
| Cherries, sweet | 8 pieces | 30 | 0 | 7 | 2 | 2 |
| Chewing gum | 1 piece | 25 | 0 | 5 | 0 | 0 |

Nutrition values for fat, carbohydrates (Cbs), protein (Prtn), and fiber (Fbr) are listed in grams per serving. Serving sizes and values are approximate.

| FOOD ITEM | Serving Size | Cal | Fat | Cbs | Prtn | Fbr |
|---|---|---|---|---|---|---|
| **C (cont.)** | | | | | | |
| Chicken, breast, w/ skin | 1/2 breast | 202 | 8 | 0 | 30 | 0 |
| Chicken, breast, w/o skin | 1/2 breast | 143 | 3 | 0 | 27 | 0 |
| Chicken, capons, boneless | 1/2 capon | 1459 | 74 | 0 | 184 | 0 |
| Chicken, capons, giblets, cooked | 1 cup | 238 | 8 | 1 | 38 | 0 |
| Chicken, cornish game hen, roasted | 1/2 bird | 336 | 24 | 0 | 29 | 0 |
| Chicken, cornish game hen, meat only | 1 bird | 295 | 9 | 0 | 51 | 0 |
| Chicken, dark meat, w/o skin | 1 cup diced | 287 | 14 | 0 | 38 | 0 |
| Chicken, drumstick, w/ skin | 1 drumstick | 118 | 6 | 0 | 14 | 0 |
| Chicken, drumstick, w/o skin | 1 drumstick | 74 | 2 | 9 | 13 | 0 |
| Chicken, leg, w/ skin | 1 leg | 265 | 15 | 0 | 30 | 0 |
| Chicken, leg, w/o skin | 1 leg | 156 | 5 | 0 | 26 | 0 |
| Chicken, light meat, w/o skin | 1 cup diced | 214 | 6 | 0 | 38 | 0 |
| Chicken, thigh, w/ skin | 1 thigh | 198 | 14 | 0 | 16 | 0 |
| Chicken, thigh, w/o skin | 1 thigh | 82 | 3 | 0 | 14 | 0 |
| Chicken, wing, w/ skin | 1 wing | 109 | 8 | 0 | 9 | 0 |
| Chicken, wing, w/o skin | 1 wing | 37 | 1 | 0 | 6 | 0 |
| Chickpeas, cooked | 1 cup | 269 | 4 | 45 | 15 | 13 |
| Chicory greens | 1 cup, chopped | 7 | 0 | 1 | 0 | 0 |
| Chicory roots | 1/2 cup | 33 | 0 | 8 | 1 | 0 |
| Chicory, witloof | 1/2 cup | 8 | 0 | 2 | 0 | 1 |
| Chili con carne w/ beans | 1 cup | 298 | 13 | 28 | 18 | 10 |
| Chili powder | 1 tsp | 8 | 0 | 1 | 0 | 1 |
| Chili w/ beans, canned | 1 cup | 287 | 14 | 31 | 15 | 11 |
| Chili w/o beans, canned | 1 cup | 194 | 7 | 18 | 17 | 3 |
| Chinese chestnuts | 1 oz. | 64 | 0 | 14 | 1 | 0 |
| Chives | 1 tbsp, chopped | 1 | 0 | 0 | 0 | 0 |
| Chocolate chip crisped rice bar | 1 bar | 115 | 4 | 21 | 1 | 1 |
| Chocolate chips | 1/4 cup | 210 | 12 | 24 | 3 | 1 |
| Chocolate milkshake, ready-to-drink | 8 fl.oz. | 181 | 5 | 26 | 8 | 1 |
| Chocolate, semi sweet bars, baking | 1 oz. | 160 | 8 | 20 | 3 | 1 |
| Chocolate, unsweetened baking squares | 1 square | 144 | 15 | 9 | 4 | 5 |
| Chorizo, pork and beef | 1 link | 273 | 23 | 1 | 15 | 0 |
| Chow mein noodles | 1 cup | 237 | 14 | 26 | 4 | 2 |
| Cinnamon, ground | 1 tsp | 6 | 0 | 2 | 0 | 1 |
| Cisco | 3 oz. | 83 | 2 | 0 | 16 | 0 |
| Citrus fruit drink, from concentrate | 8 fl.oz. | 124 | 0 | 30 | 1 | 1 |
| Clam, mixed species, raw | 1 large | 15 | 0 | 1 | 3 | 0 |
| Cloves, ground | 1 tsp | 7 | 0 | 1 | 0 | 1 |
| Cocktail mix, nonalcoholic | 1 fl.oz. | 103 | 0 | 26 | 0 | 0 |
| Cocoa mix, powder | 1 serving | 113 | 1 | 24 | 2 | 1 |

Nutrition values for fat, carbohydrates (Cbs), protein (Prtn), and fiber (Fbr)
are listed in grams per serving. Serving sizes and values are approximate.

| FOOD ITEM | Serving Size | Cal | Fat | Cbs | Prtn | Fbr |
|---|---|---|---|---|---|---|
| **C (cont.)** | | | | | | |
| Cocoa mix, powder, unsweetened | 1 tbsp | 12 | 1 | 3 | 1 | 2 |
| Coconut meat | 1 cup, shredded | 283 | 27 | 12 | 3 | 7 |
| Coconut milk | 1 cup | 552 | 57 | 13 | 6 | 5 |
| Coffee, brewed, decaf | 1 cup | 0 | 0 | 0 | 0 | 0 |
| Coffee, brewed, regular | 1 cup | 2 | 0 | 0 | 0 | 0 |
| Coffee, café au lait | 8 fl.oz. | 65 | 3 | 6 | 1 | 0 |
| Coffee, cappuccino | 8 fl.oz. | 70 | 4 | 6 | 1 | 0 |
| Coffee, espresso | 1 shot | 4 | 0 | 1 | 0 | 0 |
| Coffee, instant, decaf | 1 tsp | 0 | 0 | 0 | 0 | 0 |
| Coffee, instant, regular | 1 tsp, dry | 2 | 0 | 0 | 0 | 0 |
| Coffee, latte | 8 fl.oz. | 100 | 5 | 8 | 7 | 0 |
| Coffee, mocha | 8 fl.oz. | 180 | 2 | 32 | 11 | 1 |
| Coffee cake | 3 oz. | 230 | 7 | 38 | 4 | 4 |
| Coleslaw | 1/2 cup | 41 | 2 | 7 | 1 | 1 |
| Collards | 1 cup, chopped | 11 | 0 | 2 | 1 | 1 |
| Conch, baked or broiled | 1 cup, sliced | 165 | 2 | 2 | 33 | 0 |
| Cookies, animal crackers | 1 cookie | 22 | 1 | 4 | 0 | 0 |
| Cookies, brownies | 4 oz. | 430 | 25 | 52 | 1 | 1 |
| Cookies, butter | 1 cookie | 132 | 5 | 25 | 1 | 0 |
| Cookies, chocolate chip, deli fresh baked | 1 cookie | 275 | 15 | 38 | 0 | 1 |
| Cookies, chocolate chip, commercial | 1 cookie | 130 | 7 | 17 | 1 | 1 |
| Cookies, chocolate chip, refrigerated dough | 1 portion | 128 | 6 | 18 | 1 | 0 |
| Cookies, chocolate wafers | 1 wafer | 26 | 1 | 4 | 0 | 0 |
| Cookies, fig bars | 1 cookie | 150 | 3 | 31 | 2 | 2 |
| Cookies, fudge | 1 cookie | 73 | 1 | 16 | 1 | 1 |
| Cookies, gingersnap | 1 cookie | 29 | 1 | 5 | 0 | 0 |
| Cookies, graham, plain or honey | 2 1/2" square | 30 | 1 | 5 | 1 | 0 |
| Cookies, marshmallow w/ chocolate coating | 1 cookie | 118 | 5 | 19 | 1 | 1 |
| Cookies, molasses | 1 cookie | 138 | 4 | 24 | 2 | 0 |
| Cookies, oatmeal | 1 cookie | 67 | 3 | 10 | 1 | 0 |
| Cookies, oatmeal w/ raisins | 1 cookie | 65 | 2 | 10 | 1 | 0 |
| Cookies, oatmeal, commercial, iced | 1 cookie | 123 | 5 | 18 | 1 | 1 |
| Cookies, oatmeal, refrigerated dough | 1 portion | 68 | 3 | 10 | 1 | 0 |
| Cookies, peanut butter sandwich | 1 cookie | 67 | 3 | 9 | 1 | 0 |
| Cookies, peanut butter, refrigerated dough | 1 portion | 73 | 4 | 8 | 1 | 0 |
| Cookies, sugar | 1 cookie | 66 | 3 | 8 | 1 | 0 |
| Cookies, sugar wafers w/ cream filling | 1 wafer | 46 | 2 | 6 | 0 | 0 |
| Cookies, sugar, refrigerated dough | 1 portion | 113 | 5 | 15 | 1 | 0 |
| Cookies, vanilla wafers | 1 wafer | 28 | 1 | 4 | 0 | 0 |
| Coriander leaves | 9 sprigs | 5 | 0 | 1 | 0 | 1 |

Nutrition values for fat, carbohydrates (Cbs), protein (Prtn), and fiber (Fbr) are listed in grams per serving. Serving sizes and values are approximate.

| FOOD ITEM | Serving Size | Cal | Fat | Cbs | Prtn | Fbr |
|---|---|---|---|---|---|---|
| **C (cont.)** | | | | | | |
| Corn flour, yellow | 1 cup | 416 | 4 | 87 | 11 | 0 |
| Corn, sweet, white | 1 ear | 77 | 1 | 17 | 3 | 2 |
| Corn, sweet, yellow | 1 ear | 77 | 1 | 17 | 3 | 2 |
| Corn, sweet, white, cream style | 1 cup | 184 | 1 | 46 | 5 | 3 |
| Corn, sweet, yellow, cream style | 1 cup | 184 | 1 | 46 | 5 | 3 |
| Cornnuts | 1 oz. | 126 | 4 | 20 | 2 | 2 |
| Cornstarch | 1 cup | 488 | 0 | 117 | 0 | 1 |
| Couscous, cooked | 1 cup | 176 | 0 | 37 | 6 | 0 |
| Cowpeas (black-eyed peas), cooked | 1 cup | 160 | 1 | 34 | 5 | 8 |
| Cowpeas, catjang, cooked | 1 cup | 200 | 1 | 35 | 14 | 6 |
| Cowpeas, leafy tips | 1 cup, chopped | 10 | 0 | 2 | 2 | 0 |
| Crab, alaska king, raw | 1 leg | 144 | 1 | 0 | 32 | 0 |
| Crab, blue, canned | 1 cup | 134 | 2 | 0 | 28 | 0 |
| Crab, dungeness, cooked | 1 crab | 140 | 2 | 1 | 28 | 0 |
| Crabapples | 1 cup, sliced | 84 | 0 | 22 | 0 | 0 |
| Crackers w/ cheese filling | 6 crackers | 191 | 10 | 23 | 4 | 1 |
| Crackers w/ peanut butter filling | 6 cracker | 193 | 10 | 22 | 5 | 1 |
| Crackers, cheese, regular | 6 crackers | 312 | 16 | 36 | 6 | 2 |
| Crackers, graham | 1 cracker | 30 | 1 | 5 | 6 | 2 |
| Crackers, matzo, plain | 1 matzo | 112 | 0 | 24 | 3 | 1 |
| Crackers, matzo, whole-wheat | 1 matzo | 100 | 0 | 22 | 4 | 3 |
| Crackers, melba toast | 1 cup | 129 | 1 | 25 | 4 | 2 |
| Crackers, milk | 1 cracker | 50 | 2 | 8 | 1 | 0 |
| Crackers, regular | 1 cup, bite size | 311 | 16 | 38 | 5 | 1 |
| Crackers, rusk toast | 1 rusk | 41 | 1 | 7 | 1 | 0 |
| Crackers, rye | 1 cracker | 37 | 0 | 9 | 1 | 3 |
| Crackers, saltines | 1 cracker | 20 | 0 | 4 | 1 | 0 |
| Crackers, soda | 1 cracker | 60 | 2 | 10 | 6 | 2 |
| Crackers, wheat | 1 cracker | 9 | 0 | 1 | 0 | 0 |
| Crackers, wheat, sandwich w/ peanut butter | 1 cracker | 35 | 2 | 4 | 1 | 0 |
| Crackers, whole-wheat | 1 cracker | 18 | 1 | 3 | 0 | 0 |
| Cranberries | 1 cup, whole | 44 | 0 | 12 | 0 | 4 |
| Cranberry juice cocktail | 1 cup | 144 | 0 | 36 | 0 | 0 |
| Cranberry-apple juice | 1 cup | 174 | 0 | 44 | 0 | 0 |
| Cranberry-grape juice | 1 cup | 137 | 0 | 34 | 1 | 0 |
| Crayfish, wild, raw | 8 crayfish | 21 | 0 | 0 | 4 | 0 |
| Cream cheese | 1 tbsp | 51 | 5 | 0 | 1 | 0 |
| Cream of tartar | 1 tsp | 8 | 0 | 2 | 0 | 0 |
| Cream, half & half | 1 tbsp | 20 | 2 | 1 | 0 | 0 |
| Cream, heavy whipping | 1 cup, fluid | 821 | 88 | 7 | 5 | 0 |

Nutrition values for fat, carbohydrates (Cbs), protein (Prtn), and fiber (Fbr) are listed in grams per serving. Serving sizes and values are approximate.

| FOOD ITEM | Serving Size | Cal | Fat | Cbs | Prtn | Fbr |
|---|---|---|---|---|---|---|
| **C (cont.)** | | | | | | |
| Crêpes | 1 crêpe | 120 | 6 | 14 | 2 | 1 |
| Croissants, apple | 1 croissant | 145 | 5 | 21 | 4 | 1 |
| Croissants, butter | 1 croissant | 115 | 6 | 13 | 2 | 1 |
| Croissants, cheese | 1 croissant | 174 | 9 | 20 | 4 | 1 |
| Croutons, plain | 1 cup | 122 | 2 | 22 | 4 | 2 |
| Croutons, seasoned | 1 cup | 186 | 7 | 25 | 4 | 2 |
| Cucumber | 1 cucumber | 45 | 0 | 11 | 2 | 2 |
| Cucumber, peeled | 1 cup, sliced | 14 | 0 | 3 | 1 | 1 |
| Cumin seed | 1 tsp | 8 | 1 | 1 | 0 | 0 |
| Currants, black | 1 cup | 71 | 1 | 17 | 2 | 0 |
| Currants, red & white | 1 cup | 63 | 0 | 16 | 2 | 5 |
| Curry powder | 1 tsp | 7 | 0 | 1 | 0 | 1 |
| **D** | | | | | | |
| Dandelion greens | 1 cup, chopped | 25 | 0 | 5 | 2 | 2 |
| Danish pastry, cheese, 4 1/4" diameter | 1 pastry | 266 | 16 | 26 | 6 | 1 |
| Danish pastry, cinnamon, 4 1/4" diameter | 1 pastry | 262 | 15 | 29 | 5 | 1 |
| Danish pastry, fruit, 4 1/4" diameter | 1 pastry | 263 | 13 | 34 | 4 | 1 |
| Danish pastry, nut, 4 1/4" diameter | 1 pastry | 280 | 16 | 30 | 5 | 1 |
| Danish pastry, raspberry, 4 1/4" diameter | 1 pastry | 263 | 13 | 34 | 4 | 1 |
| Deer, ground, raw | 1 oz. | 45 | 2 | 0 | 6 | 0 |
| Deer, raw | 1 oz. | 34 | 1 | 0 | 7 | 0 |
| Doughnuts, chocolate coated or frosted | 1 doughnut | 133 | 9 | 13 | 1 | 1 |
| Doughnuts, chocolate, sugared or glazed | 1 doughnut | 250 | 12 | 34 | 3 | 1 |
| Doughnuts, french crullers | 1 cruller | 169 | 8 | 24 | 1 | 1 |
| Doughnuts, plain | 1 doughnut, stick | 219 | 12 | 26 | 3 | 1 |
| Doughnuts, wheat, sugared or glazed | 1 doughnut | 101 | 5 | 12 | 2 | 1 |
| Duck liver, raw | 1 liver | 60 | 2 | 2 | 8 | 0 |
| Duck, meat only, roasted | 1/2 duck | 444 | 25 | 0 | 52 | 0 |
| Duck, white pekin, breast w/skin, roasted | 1/2 breast | 242 | 13 | 0 | 29 | 0 |
| Duck, skinless, raw | 1/2 duck | 400 | 18 | 0 | 55 | 0 |
| Durian | 1 cup, chopped | 357 | 13 | 66 | 4 | 9 |
| **E** | | | | | | |
| Eclairs w/ chocolate glaze | 1 éclair | 293 | 18 | 27 | 7 | 1 |
| Eel, mixed species, raw | 3 oz. | 156 | 10 | 0 | 16 | 0 |
| Egg noodles, cooked | 1 cup | 213 | 2 | 40 | 8 | 2 |
| Egg substitute, liquid | 1 tbsp | 13 | 1 | 0 | 2 | 0 |
| Egg white, fried | 1 large | 92 | 7 | 0 | 6 | 0 |
| Egg white, raw | 1 large | 17 | 0 | 0 | 4 | 0 |

Nutrition values for fat, carbohydrates (Cbs), protein (Prtn), and fiber (Fbr) are listed in grams per serving. Serving sizes and values are approximate.

| FOOD ITEM | Serving Size | Cal | Fat | Cbs | Prtn | Fbr |
|---|---|---|---|---|---|---|
| **E (cont.)** | | | | | | |
| Egg yolk, raw | 1 large | 53 | 4 | 1 | 3 | 0 |
| Egg, hard-boiled | 1 cup, chopped | 211 | 14 | 2 | 17 | 0 |
| Egg, omelette | 1 large | 93 | 7 | 0 | 7 | 0 |
| Egg, poached | 1 large | 74 | 5 | 0 | 6 | 0 |
| Egg, raw | 1 large | 85 | 5.8 | 0 | 7 | 0 |
| Egg, scrambled | 1 cup | 365 | 27 | 5 | 24 | 0 |
| Eggnog | 8 fl.oz. | 343 | 19 | 34 | 10 | 0 |
| Eggplant | 1 eggplant | 110 | 10 | 26 | 5 | 16 |
| Elderberries | 1 cup | 106 | 1 | 27 | 1 | 10 |
| Elk, ground, raw | 1 oz. | 48 | 2 | 0 | 6 | 0 |
| Elk, raw | 1 oz. | 31 | 0 | 0 | 7 | 0 |
| Endive | 1 head | 87 | 1 | 17 | 6 | 16 |
| English muffins, plain | 1 muffin | 134 | 1 | 26 | 4 | 2 |
| English muffins, cinnamon-raisin | 1 muffin | 139 | 2 | 28 | 4 | 2 |
| English muffins, wheat | 1 muffin | 127 | 1 | 26 | 5 | 3 |
| English muffins, whole-wheat | 1 muffin | 134 | 1 | 27 | 6 | 4 |
| English muffins, whole-wheat/multigrain | 1 muffin | 155 | 1 | 31 | 6 | 2 |
| European chestnuts, peeled | 1 oz. | 56 | 0 | 13 | 1 | 0 |
| European chestnuts, unpeeled | 1 oz. | 60 | 1 | 13 | 3 | 2 |
| **F** | | | | | | |
| Farina, cooked | 1 cup | 112 | 0 | 24 | 3 | 1 |
| Fast food, biscuit w/ egg | 1 biscuit | 373 | 22 | 32 | 12 | 1 |
| Fast food, biscuit w/ egg & bacon | 1 biscuit | 458 | 31 | 29 | 17 | 1 |
| Fast food, biscuit w/ egg, bacon & cheese | 1 biscuit | 477 | 31 | 33 | 16 | 0 |
| Fast food, biscuit w/ sausage | 1 biscuit | 485 | 32 | 40 | 12 | 1 |
| Fast food, caramel sundae | 1 sundae | 360 | 10 | 61 | 7 | 0 |
| Fast food, cheeseburger, large, double patty | 1 sandwich | 704 | 44 | 40 | 47 | 1 |
| Fast food, cheeseburger, large, single patty | 1 sandwich | 563 | 33 | 38 | 28 | 1 |
| Fast food, corndog | 1 corndog | 460 | 19 | 56 | 17 | 1 |
| Fast food, croissant w/ egg, cheese | 1 croissant | 368 | 25 | 24 | 13 | 1 |
| Fast food, croissant w/ egg, cheese, bacon | 1 croissant | 413 | 28 | 24 | 16 | 1 |
| Fast food, croissant w/ egg, cheese, sausage | 1 croissant | 523 | 38 | 25 | 20 | 1 |
| Fast food, Danish pastry, cheese | 1 pastry | 353 | 25 | 29 | 6 | 0 |
| Fast food, Danish pastry, cinnamon | 1 pastry | 349 | 17 | 47 | 5 | 0 |
| Fast food, Danish pastry, fruit | 1 pastry | 335 | 16 | 45 | 5 | 0 |
| Fast food, fish sandwich w/ tartar sauce | 1 sandwich | 431 | 23 | 41 | 17 | 1 |
| Fast food, french toast sticks | 5 pieces | 371 | 19 | 45 | 7 | 2 |
| Fast food, fried chicken, boneless | 6 pieces | 285 | 18 | 16 | 15 | 1 |
| Fast food, hamburger, large, double patty | 1 sandwich | 540 | 27 | 40 | 34 | 2 |

Nutrition values for fat, carbohydrates (Cbs), protein (Prtn), and fiber (Fbr) are listed in grams per serving. Serving sizes and values are approximate.

| FOOD ITEM | Serving Size | Cal | Fat | Cbs | Prtn | Fbr |
|---|---|---|---|---|---|---|
| **F (cont.)** | | | | | | |
| Fast food, hamburger, large, single patty | 1 sandwich | 425 | 21 | 37 | 23 | 2 |
| Fast food, hot fudge sundae | 1 sundae | 284 | 9 | 48 | 6 | 0 |
| Fast food, hot dog w/ chili | 1 hot dog | 296 | 13 | 31 | 14 | 1 |
| Fast food, hot dog, plain | 1 hot dog | 242 | 15 | 18 | 10 | 1 |
| Fast food, McDonald's Big Mac® w/ cheese | 1 serving | 560 | 30 | 46 | 25 | 3 |
| Fast food, McDonald's Big Mac® w/o cheese | 1 serving | 495 | 25 | 43 | 23 | 3 |
| Fast food, McDonald's cheeseburger | 1 serving | 310 | 12 | 35 | 15 | 1 |
| Fast food, McDonald's Chicken McGrill® | 1 serving | 400 | 16 | 38 | 27 | 3 |
| Fast food, McDonald's Crispy Chicken | 1 serving | 500 | 23 | 50 | 24 | 3 |
| Fast food, McDonald's Filet-o-Fish® | 1 serving | 400 | 18 | 42 | 14 | 1 |
| Fast food, McDonald's french fries | 1 medium | 453 | 22 | 57 | 7 | 5 |
| Fast food, McDonald's hamburger | 1 serving | 260 | 9 | 33 | 13 | 1 |
| Fast food, McDonald's 1/4 Pounder®,cheese | 1 serving | 510 | 25 | 43 | 29 | 3 |
| Fast food, McDonald's 1/4 Pounder® | 1 serving | 420 | 18 | 40 | 24 | 3 |
| Fast food, onion rings, 8-9 rings | 1 portion | 276 | 16 | 31 | 4 | 3 |
| Fast food, strawberry sundae | 1 sundae | 268 | 8 | 45 | 6 | 0 |
| Fast food, submarine sandwich w/ cold cuts | 1 submarine 6" | 456 | 19 | 51 | 22 | 4 |
| Fast food, submarine sandwich w/ roast beef | 1 submarine 6" | 410 | 13 | 44 | 29 | 4 |
| Fast food, submarine sandwich w/ tuna | 1 submarine 6" | 584 | 28 | 55 | 30 | 4 |
| Fast food, vanilla soft-serve w/ cone | 1 cone | 164 | 6 | 24 | 4 | 0 |
| Fennel bulb | 1 cup, sliced | 27 | 0 | 6 | 1 | 3 |
| Fennel seed | 1 tbsp | 20 | 1 | 3 | 1 | 2 |
| Fenugreek seed | 1 tbsp | 36 | 1 | 7 | 3 | 3 |
| Figs | 1 medium | 37 | 0 | 10 | 0 | 2 |
| Figs, dried | 1 fig | 21 | 0 | 5 | 0 | 1 |
| Fireweed leaves | 1 cup, chopped | 24 | 1 | 4 | 1 | 2 |
| Fish oil, cod liver | 1 tbsp | 123 | 14 | 0 | 0 | 0 |
| Fish oil, herring | 1 tbsp | 123 | 14 | 0 | 0 | 0 |
| Fish oil, menhaden | 1 tbsp | 123 | 14 | 0 | 0 | 0 |
| Fish oil, salmon | 1 tbsp | 123 | 14 | 0 | 0 | 0 |
| Fish oil, sardine | 1 tbsp | 123 | 14 | 0 | 0 | 0 |
| Fish, bluefin tuna, raw | 3 oz. | 122 | 4 | 0 | 20 | 0 |
| Fish, bluefish, raw | 3 oz. | 105 | 4 | 0 | 17 | 0 |
| Fish, butterfish, raw | 3 oz. | 124 | 7 | 0 | 15 | 0 |
| Fish, carp, raw | 3 oz. | 108 | 5 | 0 | 15 | 0 |
| Fish, catfish, raw | 3 oz. | 81 | 2 | 0 | 14 | 0 |
| Fish, cod, atlantic, raw | 3 oz. | 70 | 1 | 0 | 15 | 0 |
| Fish, croaker, atlantic, raw | 3 oz. | 88 | 3 | 0 | 15 | 0 |
| Fish, flatfish, raw | 3 oz. | 77 | 1 | 0 | 16 | 0 |
| Fish, gefilte fish | 1 piece | 35 | 1 | 3 | 4 | 0 |

Nutrition values for fat, carbohydrates (Cbs), protein (Prtn), and fiber (Fbr) are listed in grams per serving. Serving sizes and values are approximate.

| FOOD ITEM | Serving Size | Cal | Fat | Cbs | Prtn | Fbr |
|---|---|---|---|---|---|---|
| **F (cont.)** | | | | | | |
| Fish, grouper, mixed species, raw | 3 oz. | 78 | 1 | 0 | 17 | 0 |
| Fish, haddock, raw | 3 oz. | 74 | 1 | 0 | 16 | 0 |
| Fish, halibut, raw | 3 oz. | 94 | 2 | 0 | 18 | 0 |
| Fish, herring, atlantic, raw | 3 oz. | 134 | 8 | 0 | 15 | 0 |
| Fish, herring, pacific, raw | 3 oz. | 166 | 12 | 0 | 14 | 0 |
| Fish, mackerel, atlantic, raw | 3 oz. | 174 | 12 | 0 | 16 | 0 |
| Fish, mackerel, king, raw | 3 oz. | 89 | 2 | 0 | 17 | 0 |
| Fish, mackerel, pacific, raw | 3 oz. | 134 | 7 | 0 | 17 | 0 |
| Fish, mackerel, spanish, raw | 3 oz. | 118 | 5 | 0 | 16 | 0 |
| Fish, milkfish, raw | 3 oz. | 126 | 6 | 0 | 18 | 0 |
| Fish, monkfish, raw | 3 oz. | 65 | 1 | 0 | 12 | 0 |
| Fish, ocean perch, atlantic, raw | 3 oz. | 80 | 1 | 0 | 16 | 0 |
| Fish, perch, mixed species, raw | 3 oz. | 77 | 1 | 0 | 17 | 0 |
| Fish, pike, northern, raw | 3 oz. | 75 | 1 | 0 | 16 | 0 |
| Fish, pollock, atlantic, raw | 3 oz. | 78 | 1 | 0 | 17 | 0 |
| Fish, pout, ocean, raw | 3 oz. | 67 | 1 | 0 | 14 | 0 |
| Fish, rainbow smelt, raw | 3 oz. | 82 | 2 | 0 | 15 | 0 |
| Fish, rockfish, pacific, raw | 3 oz. | 80 | 1 | 0 | 16 | 0 |
| Fish, roe, mixed species, raw | 1 tbsp | 20 | 1 | 0 | 3 | 0 |
| Fish, sablefish, raw | 3 oz. | 166 | 13 | 0 | 11 | 0 |
| Fish, salmon, atlantic, farmed, raw | 3 oz. | 156 | 9 | 0 | 17 | 0 |
| Fish, salmon, atlantic, wild, raw | 3 oz. | 121 | 5 | 0 | 17 | 0 |
| Fish, salmon, chinook, raw | 3 oz. | 152 | 9 | 0 | 17 | 0 |
| Fish, salmon, pink, raw | 3 oz. | 99 | 3 | 0 | 17 | 0 |
| Fish, sea bass, mixed species, raw | 3 oz. | 82 | 2 | 0 | 16 | 0 |
| Fish, seatrout, mixed species, raw | 3 oz. | 88 | 3 | 0 | 14 | 0 |
| Fish, shad, raw | 3 oz. | 167 | 12 | 0 | 14 | 0 |
| Fish, skipjack tuna, raw | 3 oz. | 88 | 1 | 0 | 19 | 0 |
| Fish, snapper, mixed species, raw | 3 oz. | 85 | 1 | 0 | 17 | 0 |
| Fish, striped bass, raw | 3 oz. | 82 | 2 | 0 | 15 | 0 |
| Fish, striped mullet | 3 oz. | 99 | 3 | 0 | 0 | 0 |
| Fish, sturgeon, mixed species, raw | 3 oz. | 89 | 3 | 0 | 14 | 0 |
| Fish, swordfish, raw | 3 oz. | 103 | 3 | 0 | 17 | 0 |
| Fish, trout, mixed species, raw | 3 oz. | 126 | 6 | 0 | 18 | 0 |
| Fish, white sucker, raw | 3 oz. | 78 | 2 | 0 | 14 | 0 |
| Fish, whitefish, raw | 3 oz. | 114 | 5 | 0 | 16 | 0 |
| Fish, wolffish, atlantic, raw | 3 oz. | 82 | 2 | 0 | 15 | 0 |
| Fish, yellowfin tuna, raw | 3 oz. | 93 | 1 | 0 | 20 | 0 |
| Fish, yellowtail, mixed species, raw | 3 oz. | 124 | 5 | 0 | 20 | 0 |
| Flan, caramel custard | 5 1/2 oz. | 303 | 12 | 43 | 4 | 0 |

Nutrition values for fat, carbohydrates (Cbs), protein (Prtn), and fiber (Fbr) are listed in grams per serving. Serving sizes and values are approximate.

| FOOD ITEM | Serving Size | Cal | Fat | Cbs | Prtn | Fbr |
|---|---|---|---|---|---|---|
| **F (cont.)** | | | | | | |
| Flaxseed | 1 tbsp | 59 | 4 | 4 | 2 | 3 |
| Flaxseed oil | 1 tbsp | 120 | 14 | 0 | 0 | 0 |
| Frankfurter | 1 serving | 151 | 13 | 2 | 5 | 0 |
| Frankfurter, beef | 1 frankfurter | 188 | 17 | 2 | 6 | 0 |
| Frankfurter, beef & pork | 1 frankfurter | 137 | 12 | 1 | 5 | 0 |
| Frankfurter, chicken | 1 frankfurter | 100 | 7 | 1 | 7 | 0 |
| Frankfurter, meat | 1 frankfurter | 151 | 13 | 2 | 5 | 0 |
| Frankfurter, meatless | 1 frankfurter | 163 | 10 | 5 | 14 | 3 |
| Frankfurter, pork | 1 frankfurter | 204 | 18 | 0 | 10 | 0 |
| Frankfurter, turkey | 1 frankfurter | 102 | 8 | 1 | 6 | 0 |
| French fries, frozen, unprepared, 18 fries | 1 serving | 170 | 7 | 28 | 3 | 3 |
| French toast, frozen, ready-to-heat | 1 piece | 126 | 4 | 19 | 4 | 1 |
| Frosting, creamy chocolate | 2 tbsp | 164 | 7 | 26 | 1 | 0 |
| Frosting, creamy vanilla | 2 tbsp | 160 | 6 | 26 | 0 | 0 |
| Frozen yogurt, chocolate, soft-serve | 1/2 cup | 115 | 4 | 18 | 3 | 2 |
| Frozen yogurt, vanilla, soft-serve | 1/2 cup | 117 | 4 | 17 | 3 | 0 |
| Fruit cocktail, canned | 1 cup | 229 | 0 | 60 | 1 | 3 |
| Fruit punch, prepared from concentrate | 8 fl.oz. | 114 | 0 | 30 | 0 | 0 |
| Fruit salad, canned in syrup | 1 cup | 186 | 0 | 49 | 1 | 3 |
| Fruit salad, canned in water | 1 cup | 74 | 0 | 19 | 1 | 3 |
| **G** | | | | | | |
| Garden cress, raw | 1 cup | 16 | 0 | 3 | 1 | 1 |
| Garlic | 1 clove | 4 | 0 | 1 | 0 | 0 |
| Garlic powder | 1 tsp | 9 | 0 | 2 | 1 | 0 |
| Gelatin dessert mix, prepared w/ water | 1/2 cup | 84 | 0 | 19 | 2 | 0 |
| Gin, 80 Proof | 1 fl.oz. | 64 | 0 | 0 | 0 | 0 |
| Ginger root | 1 tsp | 2 | 0 | 0 | 0 | 0 |
| Ginger, ground | 1 tsp | 6 | 0 | 1 | 0 | 0 |
| Ginkgo nuts | 1 oz. | 52 | 1 | 11 | 1 | 0 |
| Ginkgo nuts, dried | 1 oz. | 99 | 1 | 21 | 3 | 0 |
| Goose liver, raw | 1 liver | 125 | 4 | 6 | 15 | 0 |
| Goose, meat & skin, roasted | 1 cup chopped | 427 | 31 | 0 | 35 | 0 |
| Goose, meat only, roasted | 1 cup chopped | 340 | 18 | 0 | 41 | 0 |
| Gourd, white-flowered | 1 gourd | 108 | 0 | 26 | 5 | 0 |
| Granola bars, hard, plain | 1 bar | 118 | 5 | 16 | 3 | 1 |
| Granola bars, soft, plain | 1 bar | 126 | 5 | 19 | 2 | 1 |
| Grape juice | 8 fl.oz. | 160 | 0 | 40 | 0 | 0 |
| Grapefruit | 1/2 fruit | 50 | 0 | 12 | 1 | 3 |
| Grapefruit juice, sweetened | 8 fl.oz. | 125 | 0 | 33 | 0 | 0 |

Nutrition values for fat, carbohydrates (Cbs), protein (Prtn), and fiber (Fbr) are listed in grams per serving. Serving sizes and values are approximate.

# NUTRITION FACTS

| FOOD ITEM | Serving Size | Cal | Fat | Cbs | Prtn | Fbr |
|---|---|---|---|---|---|---|
| **G (cont.)** | | | | | | |
| Grapefruit juice, unsweetened | 8 fl.oz. | 91 | 0 | 22 | 0 | 0 |
| Grapes, canned, heavy syrup | 1 cup | 187 | 0 | 50 | 1 | 2 |
| Grapes, red or green | 1 cup | 106 | 0 | 28 | 1 | 1 |
| Gravy, mushroom, canned | 1 can | 149 | 8 | 16 | 4 | 1 |
| Gravy, au jus, canned | 1 can | 48 | 1 | 8 | 4 | 0 |
| Gravy, beef, canned | 1 can | 154 | 7 | 14 | 11 | 1 |
| Gravy, chicken, canned | 1 can | 235 | 17 | 16 | 6 | 1 |
| Gravy, turkey, canned | 1 can | 152 | 6 | 15 | 8 | 1 |
| Guacamole dip | 2 tbsp | 50 | 4 | 4 | 1 | 0 |
| Guavas | 1 fruit | 37 | 1 | 8 | 1 | 3 |
| **H** | | | | | | |
| Ham, chopped | 1 slice | 50 | 3 | 1 | 5 | 0 |
| Ham, minced | 1 slice | 55 | 4 | 0 | 3 | 0 |
| Ham, sliced | 1 slice | 46 | 2 | 1 | 5 | 0 |
| Hazlenuts, dry roasted | 1 oz. | 183 | 18 | 5 | 4 | 3 |
| Hazlenuts, blanched | 1 oz. | 178 | 17 | 5 | 4 | 3 |
| Hominy, canned, white | 1 cup | 119 | 2 | 24 | 2 | 4 |
| Hominy, canned, yellow | 1 cup | 115 | 1 | 23 | 2 | 4 |
| Honey | 1 tbsp | 64 | 0 | 17 | 0 | 0 |
| Honeydew melons | 1 cup, diced | 61 | 0 | 16 | 1 | 1 |
| Horseradish | 1 tsp | 2 | 0 | 1 | 0 | 0 |
| Hot chocolate | 8 fl.oz. | 192 | 6 | 27 | 9 | 3 |
| Hummus | 1 tbsp | 23 | 1 | 2 | 1 | 1 |
| Hush puppies | 1 hush puppy | 74 | 3 | 10 | 2 | 1 |
| **I** | | | | | | |
| Ice cream cone, rolled or sugar type | 1 cone | 40 | 0 | 8 | 1 | 0 |
| Ice cream cone, wafer or cake type | 1 cone | 17 | 0 | 3 | 0 | 0 |
| Ice cream, chocolate | 1/2 cup | 143 | 7 | 19 | 3 | 1 |
| Ice cream, strawberry | 1/2 cup | 127 | 6 | 18 | 2 | 1 |
| Ice cream, vanilla | 1/2 cup | 144 | 8 | 17 | 3 | 1 |
| Iced tea, presweetened | 8 fl.oz. | 70 | 0 | 18 | 0 | 0 |
| Iced tea, unsweetened | 8 fl.oz. | 0 | 0 | 0 | 0 | 0 |
| Italian seasoning | 1 tsp | 4 | 0 | 1 | 0 | 0 |
| **J** | | | | | | |
| Jams and preserves | 1 tbsp | 56 | 0 | 14 | 0 | 0 |
| Japanese chestnuts | 1 oz. | 44 | 0 | 10 | 1 | 0 |
| Japanese soba noodles, cooked | 1 cup | 113 | 0 | 24 | 6 | 0 |

Nutrition values for fat, carbohydrates (Cbs), protein (Prtn), and fiber (Fbr)
are listed in grams per serving. Serving sizes and values are approximate.

# NUTRITION FACTS

| FOOD ITEM | Serving Size | Cal | Fat | Cbs | Prtn | Fbr |
|---|---|---|---|---|---|---|
| **J (cont.)** | | | | | | |
| Japanese ramen noodles, packaged, dry | 1 serving | 195 | 7 | 28 | 4 | 1 |
| Jellies | 1 tbsp | 55 | 0 | 14 | 0 | 0 |
| **K** | | | | | | |
| Kale | 1 cup, chopped | 34 | 1 | 7 | 2 | 1 |
| Kiwifruit | 1 medium | 45 | 0 | 11 | 1 | 2 |
| Kumquats | 1 fruit | 13 | 0 | 3 | 0 | 1 |
| **L** | | | | | | |
| Lamb, cubed, raw | 1 oz. | 38 | 2 | 0 | 6 | 0 |
| Lamb, foreshank, raw | 1 oz. | 57 | 4 | 0 | 5 | 0 |
| Lamb, ground, raw | 1 oz. | 80 | 7 | 0 | 5 | 0 |
| Lamb, leg, shank half, raw | 1 oz. | 52 | 3 | 0 | 8 | 0 |
| Lamb, leg, sirloin half, raw | 1 oz. | 74 | 6 | 0 | 5 | 0 |
| Lamb, leg, whole, choice, raw | 1 oz. | 65 | 5 | 0 | 5 | 0 |
| Lamb, loin, choice, raw | 1 oz. | 79 | 6 | 0 | 5 | 0 |
| Lamb, rib, choice, raw | 1 oz. | 97 | 9 | 0 | 4 | 0 |
| Lamb, shoulder, arm, raw | 1 oz. | 69 | 5 | 0 | 5 | 0 |
| Lamb, shoulder, blade, raw | 1 oz. | 73 | 6 | 0 | 5 | 0 |
| Lamb, shoulder, whole, raw | 1 oz. | 69 | 5 | 0 | 5 | 0 |
| Lard | 1 tbsp | 115 | 13 | 0 | 0 | 0 |
| Leeks | 1 leek | 54 | 0 | 13 | 1 | 2 |
| Lemon juice | 1 cup | 61 | 0 | 21 | 1 | 1 |
| Lemon juice, canned or bottled | 1 tbsp | 3 | 0 | 1 | 0 | 0 |
| Lemon pepper seasoning | 1 tsp | 7 | 0 | 1 | 0 | 0 |
| Lemonade powder | 1 scoop | 102 | 0 | 27 | 0 | 0 |
| Lemonade, pink concentrate, prepared | 8 fl.oz. | 99 | 0 | 26 | 0 | 0 |
| Lemonade, white concentrate, prepared | 8 fl.oz. | 99 | 0 | 26 | 0 | 0 |
| Lemons w/ peel | 1 fruit | 22 | 0 | 12 | 1 | 5 |
| Lentils, cooked | 1 cup | 230 | 1 | 40 | 18 | 16 |
| Lentils, sprouted, raw | 1 cup | 82 | 0 | 17 | 7 | 0 |
| Lettuce, green leaf | 1 cup, shredded | 5 | 0 | 1 | 1 | 1 |
| Lettuce, iceberg | 1 cup, shredded | 10 | 0 | 2 | 1 | 1 |
| Lettuce, red leaf | 1 cup, shredded | 3 | 0 | 0 | 0 | 0 |
| Lettuce, romaine | 1 cup, shredded | 8 | 0 | 2 | 1 | 1 |
| Lime juice | 1 cup | 62 | 0 | 21 | 1 | 1 |
| Limes | 1 fruit | 20 | 0 | 7 | 1 | 2 |
| Liverwurst, pork | 1 slice | 59 | 5 | 0 | 3 | 0 |
| Lobster, northern, raw | 1 lobster | 135 | 1 | 1 | 28 | 0 |
| Luncheon meat, beef, loaved | 1 oz. | 87 | 7 | 1 | 4 | 0 |

Nutrition values for fat, carbohydrates (Cbs), protein (Prtn), and fiber (Fbr)
are listed in grams per serving. Serving sizes and values are approximate.

| FOOD ITEM | Serving Size | Cal | Fat | Cbs | Prtn | Fbr |
|---|---|---|---|---|---|---|
| **L (cont.)** | | | | | | |
| Luncheon meat, beef, thin sliced | 1 oz. | 32 | 1 | 1 | 5 | 0 |
| Luncheon meat, meatless slices | 1 slice | 26 | 2 | 1 | 3 | 0 |
| Luncheon meat, pork & chicken, minced | 1 oz. | 56 | 4 | 0 | 4 | 0 |
| Luncheon meat, pork & ham, minced | 1 oz. | 88 | 7 | 1 | 4 | 0 |
| Luncheon meat, pork or beef | 1 oz. | 99 | 9 | 1 | 4 | 0 |
| Luncheon meat, pork, canned | 1 oz. | 95 | 9 | 1 | 4 | 0 |
| Luncheon meat, pork, ham & chicken, minced | 1 oz. | 87 | 8 | 1 | 4 | 0 |
| Luncheon sausage, pork & beef | 1 oz. | 74 | 6 | 0 | 4 | 0 |
| **M** | | | | | | |
| Macadamia nuts | 1 oz. (10-12 nuts) | 203 | 22 | 4 | 2 | 2 |
| Macaroni and cheese, commercial, prepared | 1 cup | 259 | 7 | 48 | 11 | 2 |
| Macaroni, cooked | 1 cup | 221 | 1 | 43 | 8 | 3 |
| Malt drink mix, dry | 3 heaping tsp | 87 | 2 | 16 | 2 | 0 |
| Malt beverage | 8 fl.oz. | 88 | 0 | 19 | 0 | 0 |
| Mangos | 1 fruit | 135 | 1 | 35 | 1 | 4 |
| Maraschino cherries | 1 cherry | 8 | 0 | 2 | 0 | 0 |
| Margarine, fat free spread | 1 tbsp | 6 | 0 | 1 | 0 | 0 |
| Margarine, stick | 1 tbsp | 100 | 11 | 0 | 0 | 0 |
| Margarine, stick, unsalted | 1 tbsp | 102 | 11 | 0 | 0 | 0 |
| Margarine, tub | 1 tbsp | 102 | 11 | 0 | 0 | 0 |
| Martini | 1 fl.oz. | 69 | 0 | 1 | 0 | 0 |
| Mayonnaise | 1 tbsp | 57 | 5 | 4 | 0 | 0 |
| Milk, 1% low fat | 1 cup | 102 | 2 | 12 | 8 | 0 |
| Milk, 2% low fat | 1 cup | 138 | 5 | 14 | 10 | 0 |
| Milk, buttermilk, cultured, reduced fat | 1 cup | 137 | 5 | 13 | 10 | 0 |
| Milk, chocolate | 1 cup | 208 | 9 | 26 | 8 | 2 |
| Milk, dry, nonfat, instant | 1/3 cup dry | 82 | 0 | 12 | 8 | 0 |
| Milk, evaporated | 1/2 cup | 169 | 10 | 13 | 9 | 0 |
| Milk, skim or nonfat | 1 cup | 83 | 0 | 12 | 8 | 0 |
| Milk, canned, sweetened condensed | 1 cup | 982 | 27 | 167 | 24 | 0 |
| Milk, whole | 1 cup | 146 | 8 | 11 | 8 | 0 |
| Milkshake, dry mix, vanilla | 1 envelope packet | 69 | 1 | 11 | 5 | 0 |
| Millet | 1 cup | 756 | 8 | 146 | 22 | 17 |
| Miso soup | 1 cup | 36 | 1 | 5 | 2 | 1 |
| Mixed nuts | 1 cup | 814 | 71 | 35 | 24 | 12 |
| Molasses | 1 tablespoon | 58 | 0 | 15 | 0 | 0 |
| Muffins, apple bran | 1 muffin | 300 | 3 | 61 | 1 | 1 |
| Muffins, banana nut | 1 muffin | 480 | 24 | 60 | 3 | 2 |
| Muffins, blueberry | 1 muffin | 313 | 7 | 54 | 6 | 3 |

Nutrition values for fat, carbohydrates (Cbs), protein (Prtn), and fiber (Fbr) are listed in grams per serving. Serving sizes and values are approximate.

| FOOD ITEM | Serving Size | Cal | Fat | Cbs | Prtn | Fbr |
|---|---|---|---|---|---|---|
| **M (cont.)** | | | | | | |
| Muffins, chocolate chip | 1 muffin | 510 | 24 | 69 | 2 | 4 |
| Muffins, corn | 1 muffin | 345 | 10 | 58 | 7 | 4 |
| Muffins, oat bran | 1 muffin | 305 | 8 | 55 | 8 | 5 |
| Muffins, plain | 1 muffin | 242 | 9 | 36 | 4 | 2 |
| Mushrooms | 1 cup, pieces | 15 | 0 | 2 | 2 | 1 |
| Mushrooms, enoki | 1 large | 2 | 0 | 0 | 0 | 0 |
| Mushrooms, oyster | 1 large | 55 | 1 | 9 | 6 | 4 |
| Mushrooms, portabello | 1 large | 22 | 0 | 0 | 0 | 0 |
| Mushrooms, shiitake | 1 mushroom | 11 | 0 | 3 | 0 | 0 |
| Mussels, blue, raw | 1 cup | 129 | 3 | 6 | 18 | 0 |
| Mustard greens | 1 cup, chopped | 15 | 0 | 3 | 2 | 2 |
| Mustard seed, yellow | 1 tbsp | 53 | 3 | 4 | 3 | 2 |
| Mustard spinach | 1 cup, chopped | 33 | 1 | 6 | 3 | 4 |
| Mustard, prepared, yellow | 1 tsp | 3 | 0 | 0 | 0 | 0 |
| **N** | | | | | | |
| Natto (fermented soybeans) | 1 cup | 371 | 19 | 25 | 31 | 9 |
| Nectarines | 1 fruit | 60 | 0 | 15 | 2 | 2 |
| New Zealand spinach | 1 cup, chopped | 8 | 0 | 1 | 1 | 0 |
| Nutmeg, ground | 1 tsp | 12 | 1 | 0 | 1 | 1 |
| **O** | | | | | | |
| Oat bran | 1 cup | 231 | 7 | 62 | 16 | 15 |
| Oatmeal, instant, prepared w/ water | 1 cup | 129 | 2 | 22 | 5 | 4 |
| Oil, canola | 1 tbsp | 124 | 14 | 0 | 0 | 0 |
| Oil, canola & soybean | 1 tbsp | 119 | 14 | 0 | 0 | 0 |
| Oil, coconut | 1 tbsp | 116 | 14 | 0 | 0 | 0 |
| Oil, corn, peanut & olive | 1 tbsp | 124 | 14 | 0 | 0 | 0 |
| Oil, olive | 1 tbsp | 119 | 14 | 0 | 0 | 0 |
| Oil, peanut | 1 tbsp | 119 | 14 | 0 | 0 | 0 |
| Oil, sesame | 1 tbsp | 119 | 14 | 0 | 0 | 0 |
| Oil, soy | 1 tbsp | 120 | 14 | 0 | 0 | 0 |
| Oil, vegetable, almond | 1 tbsp | 120 | 14 | 0 | 0 | 0 |
| Oil, vegetable, cocoa butter | 1 tbsp | 120 | 14 | 0 | 0 | 0 |
| Oil, vegetable, coconut | 1 tbsp | 116 | 14 | 0 | 0 | 0 |
| Oil, vegetable, grapeseed | 1 tbsp | 120 | 14 | 0 | 0 | 0 |
| Oil, vegetable, hazelnut | 1 tbsp | 120 | 14 | 0 | 0 | 0 |
| Oil, vegetable, nutmeg butter | 1 tbsp | 120 | 14 | 0 | 0 | 0 |
| Oil, vegetable, palm | 1 tbsp | 120 | 14 | 0 | 0 | 0 |
| Oil, vegetable, poppyseed | 1 tbsp | 120 | 14 | 0 | 0 | 0 |

Nutrition values for fat, carbohydrates (Cbs), protein (Prtn), and fiber (Fbr)
are listed in grams per serving. Serving sizes and values are approximate.

# NUTRITION FACTS

| FOOD ITEM | Serving Size | Cal | Fat | Cbs | Prtn | Fbr |
|---|---|---|---|---|---|---|
| **O (cont.)** | | | | | | |
| Oil, vegetable, rice bran | 1 tbsp | 120 | 14 | 0 | 0 | 0 |
| Oil, vegetable, sheanut | 1 tbsp | 120 | 14 | 0 | 0 | 0 |
| Oil, vegetable, tomatoseed | 1 tbsp | 120 | 14 | 0 | 0 | 0 |
| Oil, vegetable, walnut | 1 tbsp | 120 | 14 | 0 | 0 | 0 |
| Okra | 1 cup | 31 | 0 | 7 | 2 | 3 |
| Onion powder | 1 tsp | 8 | 0 | 2 | 0 | 0 |
| Onions | 1 cup, chopped | 67 | 0 | 16 | 2 | 3 |
| Onions, sweet | 1 onion | 106 | 0 | 25 | 3 | 3 |
| Orange juice | 8 fl.oz. | 109 | 1 | 25 | 2 | 1 |
| Orange marmalade | 1 tbsp | 49 | 0 | 13 | 0 | 0 |
| Oranges | 1 large | 86 | 0 | 22 | 2 | 7 |
| Oregano, dried | 1 tsp, ground | 6 | 0 | 1 | 0 | 1 |
| Oyster, eastern, raw | 3 oz. | 50 | 1 | 5 | 4 | 0 |
| Oyster, pacific, raw | 3 oz. | 69 | 2 | 4 | 8 | 0 |
| | | | | | | |
| **P** | | | | | | |
| Pancakes, blueberry | 1 pancake | 84 | 4 | 11 | 2 | 0 |
| Pancakes, buttermilk | 1 pancake | 86 | 4 | 11 | 3 | 0 |
| Pancakes, plain, dry mix | 1 pancake | 74 | 1 | 14 | 2 | 1 |
| Papayas | 1 cup, cubed | 55 | 0 | 14 | 1 | 3 |
| Paprika | 1 tsp | 6 | 0 | 1 | 0 | 1 |
| Parsley | 1 cup | 22 | 1 | 4 | 2 | 2 |
| Parsley, dried | 1 tsp | 1 | 0 | 0 | 0 | 0 |
| Parsnips | 1 cup, sliced | 100 | 0 | 24 | 2 | 7 |
| Passion fruit | 1 fruit | 17 | 0 | 4 | 0 | 2 |
| Pasta, corn, cooked | 1 cup | 176 | 1 | 39 | 4 | 7 |
| Pasta, plain, cooked | 1 cup | 197 | 1 | 40 | 7 | 2 |
| Pasta, spinach, cooked | 1 cup | 195 | 1 | 38 | 8 | 2 |
| Pastrami, turkey | 1 oz. | 40 | 2 | 1 | 5 | 0 |
| Pâté de foie gras | 1 tbsp | 60 | 6 | 1 | 2 | 0 |
| Pâté, chicken liver, canned | 1 tbsp | 26 | 2 | 1 | 2 | 0 |
| Pâté, goose liver, canned | 1 tbsp | 60 | 6 | 1 | 2 | 0 |
| Peaches | 1 large | 61 | 0 | 15 | 1 | 2 |
| Peaches, canned | 1 cup, halved | 136 | 0 | 37 | 1 | 3 |
| Peanut butter, chunky | 2 tbsp | 188 | 16 | 7 | 8 | 3 |
| Peanut butter, smooth | 2 tbsp | 188 | 16 | 6 | 8 | 2 |
| Peanuts, dry roasted w/ salt | 1 oz. | 166 | 14 | 6 | 7 | 2 |
| Peanuts, raw | 1 oz. | 161 | 14 | 5 | 7 | 2 |
| Pears | 1 pear | 121 | 0 | 32 | 1 | 7 |
| Pears, asian | 1 pear | 116 | 1 | 29 | 1 | 10 |

Nutrition values for fat, carbohydrates (Cbs), protein (Prtn), and fiber (Fbr)
are listed in grams per serving. Serving sizes and values are approximate.

# NUTRITION FACTS

| FOOD ITEM | Serving Size | Cal | Fat | Cbs | Prtn | Fbr |
|---|---|---|---|---|---|---|
| **P (cont.)** | | | | | | |
| Pears, canned | 1 cup | 71 | 0 | 19 | 1 | 4 |
| Peas, green, fresh, cooked | 1 cup | 134 | 0 | 25 | 9 | 9 |
| Peas, green, frozen, cooked | 1 cup | 125 | 0 | 23 | 8 | 9 |
| Peas, split, cooked | 1 cup | 231 | 1 | 41 | 16 | 16 |
| Pecans | 1 oz. (20 halves) | 196 | 20 | 40 | 3 | 3 |
| Pepper, black | 1 tsp | 5 | 0 | 1 | 0 | 1 |
| Pepper, red or cayenne | 1 tsp | 6 | 0 | 1 | 0 | 1 |
| Pepperoni | 15 slices | 135 | 12 | 1 | 6 | 0 |
| Peppers, chili, green | 1/2 cup | 29 | 0 | 6 | 1 | 2 |
| Peppers, chili, red | 1/2 cup | 29 | 0 | 6 | 1 | 2 |
| Peppers, chili, sun-dried | 1 pepper | 2 | 0 | 0 | 0 | 0 |
| Peppers, jalapeno | 1 pepper | 4 | 0 | 1 | 0 | 0 |
| Peppers, sweet, green | 1 medium | 24 | 0 | 6 | 1 | 2 |
| Peppers, sweet, red | 1 medium | 31 | 0 | 7 | 1 | 2 |
| Peppers, sweet, yellow | 1 medium | 32 | 0 | 8 | 1 | 1 |
| Persimmons | 1 fruit | 32 | 0 | 8 | 0 | 0 |
| Pheasant, boneless, raw | 1/2 pheasant | 724 | 37 | 0 | 91 | 0 |
| Pheasant, breast, skinless, boneless, raw | 1/2 breast | 242 | 6 | 0 | 44 | 0 |
| Pheasant, leg, skinless, boneless, raw | 1 leg | 143 | 5 | 0 | 24 | 0 |
| Pheasant, skinless, raw | 1/2 pheasant | 468 | 13 | 0 | 83 | 0 |
| Pickle relish, sweet | 1 tbsp | 20 | 0 | 5 | 0 | 0 |
| Pickle, sour | 1 large 4" | 15 | 0 | 3 | 0 | 2 |
| Pickle, sweet | 1 large 4" | 40 | 0 | 7 | 0 | 2 |
| Pickles, dill | 1 large 4" | 24 | 0 | 6 | 1 | 2 |
| Pie crust, graham cracker, baked | 1 pie crust | 1037 | 52 | 137 | 9 | 3 |
| Pie, apple | 1 piece | 411 | 19 | 58 | 4 | 0 |
| Pie, blueberry | 1 piece | 290 | 13 | 44 | 2 | 1 |
| Pie, cherry | 1 piece | 325 | 14 | 50 | 3 | 1 |
| Pie, lemon meringue | 1 piece | 303 | 10 | 53 | 2 | 1 |
| Pie, pecan | 1 piece | 452 | 21 | 65 | 5 | 4 |
| Pie, pumpkin | 1 piece | 229 | 10 | 30 | 4 | 3 |
| Pine nuts | 1 oz. (167 nuts) | 191 | 19 | 4 | 4 | 1 |
| Pineapple | 1 fruit | 453 | 0 | 118 | 5 | 13 |
| Pineapple, canned | 1 slice | 28 | 0 | 7 | 0 | 0 |
| Pita bread, whole wheat | 1 pita | 170 | 2 | 35 | 6 | 5 |
| Pistachio nuts | 1 oz. (49 nuts) | 161 | 13 | 8 | 6 | 3 |
| Pizza, cheese | 1 slice (3.7 oz.) | 250 | 10 | 29 | 11 | 2 |
| Pizza, pepperoni | 1 slice (3.7 oz.) | 288 | 15 | 26 | 12 | 2 |
| Plantains | 1 medium | 218 | 1 | 57 | 2 | 4 |
| Plums | 1 fruit | 30 | 0 | 8 | 1 | 1 |

Nutrition values for fat, carbohydrates (Cbs), protein (Prtn), and fiber (Fbr) are listed in grams per serving. Serving sizes and values are approximate.

# NUTRITION FACTS

| FOOD ITEM | Serving Size | Cal | Fat | Cbs | Prtn | Fbr |
|---|---|---|---|---|---|---|
| **P (cont.)** | | | | | | |
| Plums, canned | 1 plum | 27 | 0 | 7 | 0 | 0 |
| Polenta | 1/2 cup | 220 | 2 | 24 | 2 | 1 |
| Pomegranates | 1 fruit | 234 | 3 | 53 | 5 | 11 |
| Popcorn cakes | 1 cake | 38 | 0 | 8 | 1 | 0 |
| Popcorn, air-popped | 1 cup | 31 | 0 | 6 | 1 | 1 |
| Popcorn, caramel-coated | 1 oz. | 122 | 4 | 22 | 1 | 2 |
| Popcorn, cheese | 1 cup | 58 | 4 | 6 | 1 | 1 |
| Popcorn, oil-popped | 1 cup | 55 | 3 | 6 | 1 | 1 |
| Popovers, dry mix | 1 oz. | 105 | 1 | 20 | 3 | 1 |
| Poppy seed | 1 tsp | 15 | 1 | 1 | 1 | 0 |
| Pork, cured, breakfast strips, cooked | 3 slices | 156 | 12 | 0 | 10 | 0 |
| Pork, cured, ham, extra lean, canned | 3 oz. | 116 | 4 | 0 | 18 | 0 |
| Pork, cured, ham, patties | 1 patty | 205 | 18 | 1 | 8 | 0 |
| Pork, cured, ham, extra lean, cooked | 3 oz. | 140 | 7 | 0 | 19 | 0 |
| Pork, cured, salt pork, raw | 1 oz. | 212 | 23 | 0 | 1 | 0 |
| Pork, fresh ground, cooked | 3 oz. | 252 | 18 | 0 | 22 | 0 |
| Pork, leg, rump half, cooked | 3 oz. | 214 | 12 | 0 | 25 | 0 |
| Pork, leg, shank half, cooked | 3 oz. | 246 | 17 | 0 | 22 | 0 |
| Pork, leg, whole, cooked | 3 oz. | 232 | 15 | 0 | 23 | 0 |
| Pork, loin, blade, cooked | 3 oz. | 275 | 21 | 0 | 20 | 0 |
| Pork, loin, center loin, cooked | 3 oz. | 199 | 11 | 0 | 22 | 0 |
| Pork, loin, center rib, cooked | 3 oz. | 214 | 13 | 0 | 23 | 0 |
| Pork, loin, sirloin, cooked | 3 oz. | 176 | 8 | 0 | 24 | 0 |
| Pork, loin, tenderloin, cooked | 3 oz. | 147 | 5 | 0 | 24 | 0 |
| Pork, loin, top loin, cooked | 3 oz. | 192 | 10 | 0 | 24 | 0 |
| Pork, loin, whole, cooked | 3 oz. | 211 | 12 | 0 | 23 | 0 |
| Pork, shoulder, arm, cooked | 3 oz. | 238 | 18 | 0 | 17 | 0 |
| Pork, shoulder, blade, cooked | 3 oz. | 229 | 16 | 0 | 20 | 0 |
| Pork, shoulder, whole, cooked | 3 oz. | 248 | 18 | 0 | 20 | 0 |
| Pork, spareribs, cooked | 3 oz. | 337 | 26 | 0 | 25 | 0 |
| Potato chips, barbecue | 1 oz. | 139 | 9 | 15 | 2 | 1 |
| Potato chips, cheese | 1 oz. | 141 | 8 | 16 | 2 | 2 |
| Potato chips, salted | 1 oz. | 152 | 10 | 15 | 2 | 1 |
| Potato chips, sour cream & onion | 1 oz. | 151 | 10 | 15 | 2 | 2 |
| Potato chips, reduced fat | 1 oz. | 134 | 6 | 19 | 2 | 2 |
| Potato chips, unsalted | 1 oz. | 152 | 10 | 15 | 2 | 1 |
| Potato flour | 1 cup | 571 | 1 | 133 | 11 | 9 |
| Potato salad | 1 cup | 358 | 21 | 28 | 7 | 3 |
| Potatoes | 1 medium | 164 | 0 | 37 | 4 | 5 |
| Potatoes, baked, w/ skin | 1 medium | 160 | 0 | 37 | 4 | 4 |

Nutrition values for fat, carbohydrates (Cbs), protein (Prtn), and fiber (Fbr)
are listed in grams per serving. Serving sizes and values are approximate.

# NUTRITION FACTS

| FOOD ITEM | Serving Size | Cal | Fat | Cbs | Prtn | Fbr |
|---|---|---|---|---|---|---|
| **P (cont.)** | | | | | | |
| Potatoes, baked, w/o skin | 1 medium | 143 | 0 | 33 | 3 | 3 |
| Potatoes, mashed | 1 cup | 237 | 9 | 35 | 4 | 3 |
| Potatoes, red | 1 medium | 153 | 0 | 34 | 4 | 4 |
| Potatoes, russet | 1 medium | 168 | 0 | 39 | 5 | 3 |
| Potatoes, scalloped | 1 cup | 211 | 9 | 26 | 7 | 5 |
| Potatoes, white | 1 medium | 149 | 0 | 34 | 4 | 5 |
| Pretzels, hard, plain, salted | 1 oz. | 108 | 1 | 22 | 3 | 1 |
| Prune juice | 8 fl.oz. | 180 | 0 | 43 | 2 | 3 |
| Pudding, banana | 1/2 cup | 154 | 3 | 29 | 4 | 0 |
| Pudding, chocolate | 1/2 cup | 154 | 3 | 28 | 5 | 0 |
| Pudding, coconut cream | 1/2 cup | 157 | 3 | 28 | 4 | 0 |
| Pudding, lemon | 1/2 cup | 157 | 3 | 30 | 4 | 0 |
| Pudding, rice | 1/2 cup | 163 | 2 | 31 | 5 | 0 |
| Pudding, tapioca | 1/2 cup | 154 | 2 | 29 | 4 | 0 |
| Pudding, vanilla | 1/2 cup | 148 | 3 | 27 | 4 | 0 |
| Pumpkin | 1 cup | 30 | 0 | 8 | 1 | 1 |
| Pumpkin pie mix | 1 cup | 281 | 0 | 71 | 3 | 22 |
| Pumpkin, canned | 1 cup | 83 | 1 | 20 | 3 | 7 |
| **R** | | | | | | |
| Rabbit, cooked | 3 oz. | 167 | 7 | 0 | 25 | 0 |
| Radicchio | 1 cup, shredded | 9 | 0 | 2 | 1 | 0 |
| Radishes | 1 cup, sliced | 19 | 0 | 4 | 1 | 2 |
| Raisins | 1 1/2 oz. | 129 | 0 | 34 | 1 | 2 |
| Raisins, golden | 1 1/2 oz. | 130 | 0 | 34 | 1 | 2 |
| Raspberries | 1 cup | 64 | 1 | 15 | 2 | 8 |
| Rhubarb | 1 cup, diced | 26 | 0 | 6 | 1 | 2 |
| Rice cakes, brown rice, corn | 1 cake | 35 | 0 | 7 | 1 | 0 |
| Rice cakes, brown rice, multigrain | 1 cake | 35 | 0 | 7 | 1 | 0 |
| Rice cakes, brown rice, plain | 1 cake | 35 | 0 | 7 | 1 | 0 |
| Rice, brown, cooked | 1 cup | 218 | 2 | 46 | 5 | 4 |
| Rice, white, cooked | 1 cup | 242 | 0 | 53 | 4 | 1 |
| Rice, wild | 1 cup | 166 | 1 | 35 | 7 | 3 |
| Rolls, dinner | 1 roll | 136 | 3 | 23 | 4 | 1 |
| Rolls, dinner, wheat | 1 roll | 76 | 2 | 13 | 2 | 1 |
| Rolls, dinner, whole-wheat | 1 roll | 114 | 2 | 22 | 4 | 3 |
| Rolls, french | 1 roll | 119 | 2 | 22 | 4 | 0 |
| Rolls, hamburger or hotdog | 1 roll | 120 | 2 | 21 | 4 | 1 |
| Rolls, hard (incl. kaiser) | 1 roll | 126 | 2 | 23 | 4 | 1 |
| Rolls, pumpernickel | 1 roll | 119 | 1 | 23 | 5 | 2 |

Nutrition values for fat, carbohydrates (Cbs), protein (Prtn), and fiber (Fbr)
are listed in grams per serving. Serving sizes and values are approximate.

| FOOD ITEM | Serving Size | Cal | Fat | Cbs | Prtn | Fbr |
|---|---|---|---|---|---|---|
| **R (cont.)** | | | | | | |
| Rosemary | 1 tsp | 1 | 0 | 0 | 0 | 0 |
| Rosemary, dried | 1 tsp | 4 | 0 | 1 | 0 | 1 |
| Rum, 80 proof | 1 fl.oz. | 64 | 0 | 0 | 0 | 0 |
| Rutabagas | 1 cup, cubed | 50 | 0 | 11 | 2 | 4 |
| Rye | 1 cup | 566 | 4 | 118 | 56 | 25 |
| Rye flour, dark | 1 cup | 415 | 3 | 88 | 18 | 29 |
| Rye flour, light | 1 cup | 374 | 1 | 82 | 9 | 15 |
| Rye flour, medium | 1 cup | 361 | 2 | 79 | 10 | 15 |
| | | | | | | |
| **S** | | | | | | |
| Sage, ground | 1 tsp | 2 | 0 | 0 | 0 | 0 |
| Sake | 1 fl.oz. | 39 | 0 | 2 | 0 | 0 |
| Salad dressing, 1000 island | 1 tbsp | 58 | 6 | 2 | 0 | 0 |
| Salad dressing, bacon & tomato | 1 tbsp | 49 | 5 | 0 | 0 | 0 |
| Salad dressing, blue cheese | 1 tbsp | 77 | 8 | 1 | 1 | 0 |
| Salad dressing, caesar | 1 tbsp | 78 | 9 | 1 | 0 | 0 |
| Salad dressing, coleslaw | 1 tbsp | 61 | 5 | 4 | 0 | 0 |
| Salad dressing, french | 1 tbsp | 71 | 7 | 2 | 0 | 0 |
| Salad dressing, honey dijon | 1 tbsp | 58 | 5 | 3 | 1 | 1 |
| Salad dressing, italian | 1 tbsp | 43 | 4 | 2 | 0 | 0 |
| Salad dressing, mayo-based | 1 tbsp | 57 | 5 | 4 | 0 | 0 |
| Salad dressing, mayonnaise | 1 tbsp | 103 | 12 | 0 | 0 | 0 |
| Salad dressing, peppercorn | 1 tbsp | 76 | 8 | 1 | 0 | 0 |
| Salad dressing, ranch | 1 tbsp | 73 | 8 | 1 | 0 | 0 |
| Salad dressing, russian | 1 tbsp | 76 | 8 | 2 | 0 | 0 |
| Salad, chicken | 6 oz. | 420 | 33 | 11 | 29 | 2 |
| Salad, egg | 6 oz. | 300 | 23 | 14 | 20 | 1 |
| Salad, prima pasta | 6 oz. | 360 | 30 | 18 | 5 | 3 |
| Salad, seafood w/ crab & shrimp | 6 oz. | 420 | 34 | 20 | 0 | 0 |
| Salad, tuna | 6 oz. | 450 | 36 | 14 | 16 | 0 |
| Salami, cooked, turkey | 1 oz. | 38 | 2 | 0 | 4 | 0 |
| Salami, dry, pork or beef | 3 slices | 104 | 8 | 1 | 6 | 0 |
| Salami, italian pork | 1 oz. | 119 | 10 | 0 | 6 | 0 |
| Salsa, w/ oil | 2 tbsp | 40 | 3 | 8 | 0 | 0 |
| Salsa, w/o oil | 2 tbsp | 15 | 0 | 4 | 0 | 0 |
| Salt | 1 tbsp | 0 | 0 | 0 | 0 | 0 |
| Sauce, alfredo | 1/4 cup | 120 | 11 | 3 | 15 | 2 |
| Sauce, barbecue | 1 cup | 375 | 1 | 91 | 0 | 2 |
| Sauce, cheese | 1 cup | 479 | 36 | 13 | 25 | 0 |
| Sauce, cranberry | 1 cup | 418 | 0 | 108 | 1 | 3 |

Nutrition values for fat, carbohydrates (Cbs), protein (Prtn), and fiber (Fbr) are listed in grams per serving. Serving sizes and values are approximate.

| FOOD ITEM | Serving Size | Cal | Fat | Cbs | Prtn | Fbr |
|---|---|---|---|---|---|---|
| **S (cont.)** | | | | | | |
| Sauce, hollandaise | 1 cup | 62 | 2 | 10 | 2 | 0 |
| Sauce, honey mustard | 1 tbsp | 30 | 1 | 5 | 0 | 0 |
| Sauce, marinara | 1 cup | 185 | 6 | 28 | 5 | 1 |
| Sauce, salsa | 1 cup | 70 | 0 | 16 | 4 | 4 |
| Sauce, soy | 1 tbsp | 10 | 0 | 0 | 0 | 0 |
| Sauce, steak | 1 tbsp | 25 | 0 | 6 | 0 | 0 |
| Sauce, teriyaki | 1 tbsp | 15 | 0 | 2 | 17 | 0 |
| Sauce, tomato chili | 1 cup | 284 | 1 | 54 | 7 | 16 |
| Sauce, worcestershire | 1 cup | 214 | 0 | 54 | 0 | 0 |
| Sauerkraut | 1/2 cup | 25 | 0 | 5 | 1 | 4 |
| Sausage, italian pork, raw | 1 link | 391 | 35 | 1 | 16 | 0 |
| Sausage, pork | 1 link | 85 | 7 | 0 | 4 | 0 |
| Sausage, smoked linked, pork | 1 link | 265 | 22 | 1 | 15 | 0 |
| Sausage, turkey | 1 oz. | 55 | 3 | 0 | 7 | 0 |
| Savory, ground | 1 tsp | 4 | 0 | 1 | 0 | 1 |
| Scallops | 1 scallop | 26 | 0 | 1 | 5 | 0 |
| Seaweed, dried | 1 oz. | 81 | 2 | 7 | 16 | 1 |
| Sesame seeds, dried | 1 tbsp | 52 | 5 | 2 | 2 | 1 |
| Shallots | 1 tbsp, chopped | 7 | 0 | 2 | 0 | 0 |
| Shortening | 1 tbsp | 113 | 13 | 0 | 0 | 0 |
| Shrimp, mixed species, raw | 1 medium piece | 6 | 0 | 0 | 1 | 0 |
| Snacks, cheese puffs or twists | 1 oz. | 157 | 10 | 15 | 2 | 0 |
| Soda, club | 12 fl.oz. | 0 | 0 | 0 | 0 | 0 |
| Soda, cream | 12 fl.oz. | 189 | 0 | 49 | 0 | 0 |
| Soda, diet cola | 12 fl.oz. | 7 | 0 | 0 | 0 | 0 |
| Soda, ginger ale | 12 fl.oz. | 124 | 0 | 32 | 0 | 0 |
| Soda, lemon-lime | 12 fl.oz. | 151 | 0 | 38 | 0 | 0 |
| Soda, regular, w/ caffeine | 12 fl.oz. | 155 | 0 | 40 | 0 | 0 |
| Soda, regular, w/o caffeine | 12 fl.oz. | 207 | 0 | 53 | 0 | 0 |
| Soda, root beer | 12 fl.oz. | 152 | 0 | 39 | 0 | 0 |
| Soda, tonic water | 12 fl.oz. | 124 | 0 | 32 | 0 | 0 |
| Soup, beef broth | 1 cup | 17 | 1 | 0 | 3 | 0 |
| Soup, beef stroganoff | 1 cup | 235 | 11 | 22 | 12 | 1 |
| Soup, beef vegetable | 1/2 cup | 82 | 2 | 13 | 3 | 1 |
| Soup, chicken broth | 1 cup | 39 | 1 | 1 | 5 | 0 |
| Soup, chicken noodle | 1/2 cup | 75 | 2 | 9 | 4 | 1 |
| Soup, chicken vegetable | 1/2 cup | 75 | 3 | 9 | 4 | 1 |
| Soup, chicken w/ dumplings | 1/2 cup | 96 | 6 | 6 | 6 | 1 |
| Soup, clam chowder | 1 cup | 134 | 3 | 18 | 7 | 3 |
| Soup, cream of chicken | 1 cup | 223 | 15 | 18 | 6 | 0 |

Nutrition values for fat, carbohydrates (Cbs), protein (Prtn), and fiber (Fbr) are listed in grams per serving. Serving sizes and values are approximate.

| FOOD ITEM | Serving Size | Cal | Fat | Cbs | Prtn | Fbr |
|---|---|---|---|---|---|---|
| **S (cont.)** | | | | | | |
| Soup, cream of mushroom | 1 cup | 204 | 14 | 16 | 4 | 0 |
| Soup, cream of potato | 1 cup | 149 | 6 | 17 | 6 | 1 |
| Soup, minestrone | 1/2 cup | 82 | 3 | 11 | 4 | 1 |
| Soup, split-pea w/ham | 1 cup | 379 | 9 | 56 | 21 | 5 |
| Soup, tomato | 1 cup | 161 | 6 | 22 | 6 | 3 |
| Soup, vegetarian | 1 cup | 72 | 2 | 12 | 2 | 1 |
| Sour cream | 1 tbsp | 26 | 2.5 | 1 | 0 | 0 |
| Sour cream, fat free | 1 tbsp | 9 | 0 | 2 | 0 | 0 |
| Sour cream, reduced fat | 1 tbsp | 22 | 2 | 1 | 1 | 0 |
| Soy milk | 1 cup | 127 | 5 | 12 | 11 | 3 |
| Soy protein isolate | 1 oz. | 96 | 1 | 2 | 23 | 2 |
| Soybeans, green, cooked | 1 cup | 254 | 12 | 20 | 22 | 7 |
| Soybeans, nuts, roasted | 1/4 cup | 194 | 9 | 14 | 17 | 3 |
| Soyburger | 1 patty | 125 | 4 | 9 | 13 | 3 |
| Spaghetti, cooked | 1 cup | 197 | 1 | 40 | 7 | 2 |
| Spaghetti, spinach, cooked | 1 cup | 182 | 1 | 37 | 6 | 2 |
| Spaghetti, whole-wheat, cooked | 1 cup | 174 | 1 | 37 | 7 | 6 |
| Spinach | 1 cup | 7 | 0 | 1 | 1 | 1 |
| Squab, boneless, raw | 1 squab | 585 | 47 | 0 | 37 | 0 |
| Squab, skinless, raw | 1 squab | 239 | 13 | 0 | 29 | 0 |
| Squash, summer | 1 cup, sliced | 18 | 0 | 4 | 1 | 1 |
| Squash, winter | 1 cup, cubed | 39 | 0 | 10 | 1 | 2 |
| Squid, mixed species, raw | 1 oz. | 26 | 0 | 1 | 4 | 0 |
| Stock, beef | 1 cup | 31 | 0 | 3 | 5 | 0 |
| Stock, chicken | 1 cup | 86 | 3 | 9 | 6 | 0 |
| Stock, fish | 1 cup | 40 | 2 | 0 | 5 | 0 |
| Strawberries | 1 cup | 49 | 1 | 12 | 1 | 3 |
| Succotash | 1 oz. | 28 | 0 | 5 | 1 | 1 |
| Sugar, brown | 1 tsp | 12 | 0 | 3 | 0 | 0 |
| Sugar, granulated | 1 tsp | 16 | 0 | 4 | 0 | 0 |
| Sugar, maple | 1 tsp | 11 | 0 | 3 | 0 | 0 |
| Sugar, powdered | 1 tsp | 10 | 0 | 3 | 0 | 0 |
| Sunflower seeds | 1 tbsp | 47 | 4 | 2 | 2 | 1 |
| Sweet potato | 1 cup, cubed | 114 | 0 | 27 | 2 | 4 |
| Syrup, chocolate | 1 tbsp | 67 | 2 | 12 | 1 | 1 |
| Syrup, dark corn | 1 tbsp | 57 | 0 | 16 | 0 | 0 |
| Syrup, grenadine | 1 tbsp | 53 | 0 | 13 | 0 | 0 |
| Syrup, light corn | 1 tbsp | 59 | 0 | 16 | 0 | 0 |
| Syrup, maple | 1 tbsp | 52 | 0 | 13 | 0 | 0 |
| Syrup, pancake | 1 tbsp | 47 | 0 | 12 | 0 | 0 |

Nutrition values for fat, carbohydrates (Cbs), protein (Prtn), and fiber (Fbr)
are listed in grams per serving. Serving sizes and values are approximate.

# NUTRITION FACTS

| FOOD ITEM | Serving Size | Cal | Fat | Cbs | Prtn | Fbr |
|---|---|---|---|---|---|---|
| **T** | | | | | | |
| Taco shell, hard | 1 shell | 55 | 3 | 6 | 1 | 1 |
| Tangerines | 1 large | 52 | 0 | 13 | 1 | 2 |
| Tarragon, dried | 1 tsp | 2 | 0 | 0 | 0 | 0 |
| Tea, instant | 1 cup | 2 | 0 | 0 | 0 | 0 |
| Thyme | 1 tsp | 1 | 0 | 0 | 0 | 0 |
| Thyme, dried | 1 tsp | 3 | 0 | 1 | 0 | 0 |
| Tofu, firm | 1/2 cup | 183 | 11 | 5 | 20 | 3 |
| Tofu, fried | 1 piece | 35 | 3 | 1 | 2 | 1 |
| Tofu, soft | 1/2 cup | 76 | 5 | 2 | 8 | 0 |
| Tomato juice, canned, with salt | 6 fl.oz. | 31 | 0 | 8 | 1 | 1 |
| Tomato juice, canned, without salt | 6 fl.oz. | 30 | 0 | 8 | 1 | 1 |
| Tomato paste, canned | 1/2 cup | 107 | 1 | 25 | 6 | 6 |
| Tomato sauce, canned | 1 cup | 78 | 1 | 18 | 3 | 4 |
| Tomatoes, canned, crushed | 1 cup | 82 | 1 | 19 | 4 | 5 |
| Tomatoes, green | 1 cup, chopped | 41 | 0 | 9 | 2 | 2 |
| Tomatoes, orange | 1 cup, chopped | 25 | 0 | 5 | 2 | 1 |
| Tomatoes, red | 1 cup, chopped | 32 | 0 | 7 | 2 | 2 |
| Tomatoes, sun-dried | 1 cup, chopped | 139 | 2 | 30 | 8 | 7 |
| Toppings, butterscotch or caramel | 2 tbsp | 103 | 0 | 27 | 1 | 0 |
| Toppings, marshmallow cream | 2 tbsp | 132 | 0 | 32 | 0 | 0 |
| Toppings, nuts in syrup | 2 tbsp | 184 | 9 | 24 | 2 | 1 |
| Toppings, pineapple | 2 tbsp | 106 | 0 | 28 | 0 | 0 |
| Toppings, strawberry | 2 tbsp | 107 | 0 | 28 | 0 | 0 |
| Tortilla chips, plain | 1 oz. | 142 | 7 | 18 | 2 | 2 |
| Tortilla, corn | 1 tortilla | 45 | 1 | 9 | 2 | 3 |
| Tortilla, flour | 1 tortilla | 146 | 3 | 25 | 4 | 0 |
| Trail mix | 1/4 cup | 173 | 11 | 17 | 5 | 3 |
| Turkey, deli sliced, white meat | 1 oz. | 30 | 1 | 1 | 5 | 0 |
| Turkey, back, skinless, boneless, raw | 1/2 back | 180 | 5 | 0 | 31 | 0 |
| Turkey, breast, boneless, raw | 1/2 breast | 433 | 3 | 0 | 96 | 0 |
| Turkey, breast, skinless, boneless, raw | 1/2 breast | 161 | 3 | 0 | 30 | 0 |
| Turkey, dark meat, boneless, raw | 1/2 turkey | 686 | 26 | 0 | 107 | 0 |
| Turkey, dark meat, skinless, boneless, raw | 1/2 turkey | 532 | 13 | 0 | 98 | 0 |
| Turkey, leg, boneless, raw | 1 leg | 232 | 13 | 0 | 27 | 0 |
| Turkey, leg, skinless, boneless, raw | 1 leg | 192 | 8 | 0 | 28 | 0 |
| Turkey, wing, boneless, raw | 1 wing | 204 | 10 | 0 | 27 | 0 |
| Turkey, wing, skinless, boneless, raw | 1 wing | 95 | 1 | 0 | 20 | 0 |
| Turkey, young hen, back, boneless, raw | 1/2 back | 216 | 16 | 0 | 27 | 0 |
| Turkey, young hen, breast, boneless, raw | 1/2 breast | 194 | 8 | 0 | 29 | 0 |
| Turkey, young hen, dark meat, boneless, raw | 1/2 turkey | 1056 | 40 | 0 | 163 | 0 |

Nutrition values for fat, carbohydrates (Cbs), protein (Prtn), and fiber (Fbr)
are listed in grams per serving. Serving sizes and values are approximate.

| FOOD ITEM | Serving Size | Cal | Fat | Cbs | Prtn | Fbr |
|---|---|---|---|---|---|---|
| **T (cont.)** | | | | | | |
| Turkey, young hen, leg, boneless, raw | 1 leg | 213 | 13 | 0 | 27 | 0 |
| Turkey, young hen, wing, boneless, raw | 1 wing | 238 | 13 | 0 | 27 | 0 |
| Turkey, young tom, back, boneless, raw | 1/2 back | 180 | 5 | 0 | 31 | 0 |
| Turkey, young tom, breast, boneless, raw | 1/2 breast | 194 | 8 | 0 | 29 | 0 |
| Turkey, young tom, dark meat, boneless, raw | 1/2 turkey | 1884 | 63 | 0 | 307 | 0 |
| Turkey, young tom, leg, boneless, raw | 1 leg | 213 | 11 | 0 | 28 | 0 |
| Turkey, young tom, wing, boneless, raw | 1 wing | 238 | 13 | 0 | 27 | 0 |
| Turnip greens | 1 cup, chopped | 18 | 0 | 4 | 1 | 2 |
| Turnips | 1 cup, cubed | 36 | 0 | 8 | 1 | 2 |
| **V** | | | | | | |
| Vanilla extract | 1 tbsp | 37 | 0 | 2 | 0 | 0 |
| Veal, breast, raw | 1 oz. | 59 | 4 | 0 | 5 | 0 |
| Veal, cubed, raw | 1 oz. | 31 | 1 | 0 | 6 | 0 |
| Veal, ground, raw | 1 oz. | 41 | 2 | 0 | 6 | 0 |
| Veal, leg, raw | 1 oz. | 33 | 1 | 0 | 6 | 0 |
| Veal, loin, raw | 1 oz. | 46 | 3 | 0 | 5 | 0 |
| Veal, rib, raw | 1 oz. | 46 | 3 | 0 | 5 | 0 |
| Veal, shank, raw | 1 oz. | 32 | 1 | 0 | 5 | 0 |
| Veal, shoulder, arm, raw | 1 oz. | 37 | 2 | 0 | 6 | 0 |
| Veal, shoulder, blade, raw | 1 oz. | 37 | 2 | 0 | 6 | 0 |
| Veal, shoulder, whole, raw | 1 oz. | 37 | 2 | 0 | 6 | 0 |
| Veal, sirloin, raw | 1 oz. | 43 | 2 | 0 | 5 | 0 |
| Vegetable juice | 8 fl.oz. | 50 | 0 | 12 | 2 | 2 |
| Vinegar | 1 tbsp | 2 | 0 | 1 | 0 | 0 |
| **W** | | | | | | |
| Waffles, plain | 1 waffle | 218 | 11 | 25 | 6 | 0 |
| Walnuts | 1 oz. (14 halves) | 185 | 19 | 4 | 4 | 2 |
| Wasabi root | 1 cup, sliced | 142 | 1 | 31 | 6 | 10 |
| Water chestnuts, chinese | 1/2 cup, sliced | 60 | 0 | 15 | 1 | 2 |
| Watercress | 1 cup, chopped | 4 | 0 | 0 | 1 | 0 |
| Watermelon | 1 cup, diced | 46 | 0 | 12 | 1 | 1 |
| Wheat bran | 1 cup | 125 | 3 | 37 | 9 | 25 |
| Wheat flour, whole grain | 1 cup | 407 | 2 | 87 | 16 | 15 |
| Wheat germ | 1 cup | 414 | 11 | 60 | 27 | 15 |
| Whipped cream | 1 cup | 154 | 13 | 8 | 2 | 0 |
| Wine, cooking | 1 tsp | 2 | 0 | 0 | 0 | 0 |
| Wine, red | 3-1/2 oz. glass | 74 | 0 | 2 | 0 | 0 |
| Wine, rose | 3-1/2 oz. glass | 73 | 0 | 1 | 0 | 0 |

Nutrition values for fat, carbohydrates (Cbs), protein (Prtn), and fiber (Fbr) are listed in grams per serving. Serving sizes and values are approximate.

# NUTRITION FACTS

| FOOD ITEM | Serving Size | Cal | Fat | Cbs | Prtn | Fbr |
|---|---|---|---|---|---|---|
| **W (cont.)** | | | | | | |
| Wine, white | 3-1/2 oz. glass | 70 | 0 | 1 | 0 | 0 |
| | | | | | | |
| **Y** | | | | | | |
| Yam | 1 cup, cubed | 177 | 0 | 42 | 2 | 6 |
| Yeast, active, dry | 1 tsp | 12 | 0 | 2 | 2 | 1 |
| Yogurt, fruit, low fat | 8 oz. container | 118 | 0 | 24 | 6 | 0 |
| Yogurt, fruit, whole milk | 8 oz. container | 250 | 6 | 38 | 9 | 0 |
| Yogurt, plain, lowfat | 8 oz. container | 110 | 4 | 7 | 8 | 0 |
| Yogurt, plain, whole milk | 8 oz. container | 138 | 7 | 11 | 12 | 0 |
| | | | | | | |
| **Z** | | | | | | |
| Zucchini | 1 medium | 31 | 0 | 7 | 2 | 2 |

Nutrition values for fat, protein (Prtn), carbohydrates (Cbs), and fiber (Fbr) are listed in grams per serving.  Serving sizes and values are approximate.

## Tell Us Your Success Story!

Did you lose weight, break bad habits, and make new healthy ones with this book? We love when our readers share their weight-loss success stories with us!

Please tell us your story, your initial weight and measurements, your expectations for this diet and fitness program, etc. Tell us what you liked or didn't like about this book, and what you found useful or wished we had included. Now, tell us how you feel with your new slimmer and healthier body. Or maybe you want to share your advice for others who are struggling with their weight.

Please include the following information:

- Your name:
- Phone number:
- E-mail:
- Your story!
- Before and After photos, if possible

Please email this information to info@WSPublishingGroup.com or send a letter to WS Publishing Group, 15373 Innovation Drive, Suite 360; San Diego, CA 92128.

# Notes:

# Notes:

# Notes:

# Notes:

# Notes:

# Notes:

# Interval Timer
## Workout & Fitness **PRO**

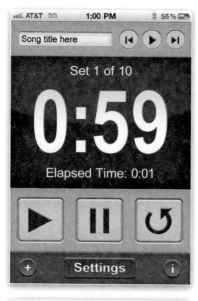

**Working out has never been easier!** The *Interval Timer: Workout & Fitness PRO* keeps you motivated and makes exercise fun.

**Special Features:**
- Large, easy-to-read display & buttons
- Tracks number of sets performed
- Shows elapsed time and rest periods
- Gives multiple cue options for sets and rest periods
- Plays music from your iTunes library

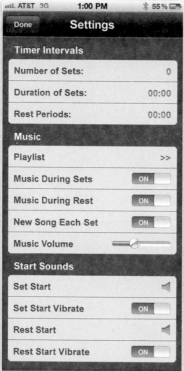

**So easy to use:**
1) Enter the number of sets you desire, as well as the length of time for each set and rest period.

2) Select a custom ringtone or set your iPhone to vibrate to cue you at the start of each set and/or rest period.

Or, play your favorite music from your iTunes Library. You can even choose a new song to start off each set!

Search the iTunes App store for
**Interval Timer Workout & Fitness PRO**